The Nutri/System® Flavor Set-Point® Weight-Loss Cookbook

THE Nutri/System® Flavor Set-Point® Weight-Loss Cookbook

Susan S. Schiffman, Ph.D., and Joan Scobey

Recipes by Robin Rifkin

LITTLE, BROWN AND COMPANY

Boston • Toronto • London

Nutri/System and Flavor Set-Point are
registered trademarks of Nutri/System, Inc.
Premier is a trademark of Nutri/System, Inc.

Before embarking on any weight-loss or exercise
program, including this one, it is advisable to
consult with your physician.

Library of Congress Cataloging-in-Publication Data

Schiffman, Susan S.
  The Nutri/System Flavor Set-Point weight-loss
cookbook / Susan S. Schiffman, and Joan Scobey;
recipes by Robin Rifkin.
     p.   cm.
  ISBN 0-316-77311-5 (HC)
  ISBN 0-316-77341-7 (PB)
  1. Reducing diets—Recipes.   I. Scobey, Joan.
II. Rifkin, Robin.   III. Title.
RM222.2.S275   1990
641.5'635—dc20   89-37278

                HC: 10 9 8 7
                PB: 10 9 8 7 6 5 4 3

      Text design by Joyce C. Weston

                    MV NY

      *Published simultaneously in Canada
      by Little, Brown & Company (Canada) Limited*

PRINTED IN THE UNITED STATES OF AMERICA

Contents

II. A Primer of Weight-Control Cooking   43

III. The Recipes   59

IV. Menu Planner   301

Introduction

SINCE 1971, millions of people have successfully achieved weight loss on the Nutri/System Weight Loss Program. And it's a record we're proud of! That's why we've developed *The Nutri/System Flavor Set-Point Weight-Loss Cookbook*—to introduce millions of others to the basic principles of our weight-loss program and help them prepare high-flavor, low-calorie, nutritious meals in their own homes.

The Nutri/System Program is built on a nutritionally balanced meal plan that tastes good, provides lots of flavor and texture, and reduces caloric intake. This meal plan is based on the Flavor Set-Point Theory. According to the Flavor Set-Point Theory, overweight people need greatly intensified flavor and varied texture in their food to feel fully satisfied with what they've eaten. By *satisfying* client needs with a wide range of *real* food choices and Flavor Enhancers, the Nutri/System Program spells successful weight control for millions of Nutri/System clients.

What Is the Flavor Set-Point Theory?

The recipes in this cookbook are based on the Flavor Set-Point Theory that was developed by Susan S. Schiffman, Ph.D., Professor of Medical Psychology at Duke University Medical Center and Director of the Weight Loss Unit. After years of research in nutrition and psychology, Dr. Schiffman concludes that all of us, whether thin or overweight, have a specific requirement—a "set-point"—for flavor and texture in our food. And to feel *satisfied* with what we eat and drink, we must reach that set-point level.

Dr. Schiffman also observed that overweight people have an exaggerated flavor and texture set-point. She realized that when the flavor and texture of their food are intense and varied enough, they feel *satisfied* with a low-calorie diet, are better able to control their food intake, and thus lose or control their weight.

Dr. Schiffman's Flavor Set-Point Theory may sound simple, but it is an important finding: When dieters feel fully satisfied with the taste and texture of their meals, they are less tempted to binge and gain back lost weight. By satisfying their food cravings, these dieters are no longer "restrained eaters"—potential bingers who compensate for feeling deprived by eating uncontrollably as soon as their restraint fails.

The result? They are more successful at controlling their weight. That's why Nutri/System invited Dr. Schiffman to join our National Health Sciences Advisory Board in 1985: to help us incorporate her research in the fields of obesity, weight control, and the biochemistry of foods into our weight-loss program.

Some Background on the Nutri/System Program

The 1983 International Congress on Obesity has established standards for professional weight-control programs: low-calorie meal plans, behavior and nutrition counseling, and exercise. The Nutri/System Weight Loss Program is designed to meet those standards by providing clients with structured 1100–1500 calorie meal plans, along with the nutritional and psychological support they need to *control* their weight.

The Nutri/System Weight Loss Program takes all aspects of weight control very seriously. Founded in 1971, we continually follow scientific investigations and advances in the fields of nutrition, obesity, health, and fitness, and update our program to reflect the very latest research in these areas.

Our Nutri/System staff professionals work closely with our National Health Sciences Advisory Board, an active panel of distinguished scientists. In addition to Dr. Schiffman, who advises us on the psychology and biochemistry of weight control, we have the counsel of Judith Rodin, Ph.D., Professor of Psychiatry and Professor of Medicine, Yale University; Peter D. Wood, D.Sc., Ph.D., Professor of Medical Research, Stanford University School of Medicine; Michael

Feuerstein, Ph.D., Director of Behavioral Medicine Programs, University of Rochester School of Medicine; Jay A. Winsten, Ph.D., Director of the Harvard Center of Health Communication and Assistant Dean, Harvard School of Public Health; Bonnie Spring, Ph.D., Professor of Psychology, University of Health Sciences, Chicago Medical School.

Let me tell you a little about the Nutri/System Weight Loss Program. At our nearly 1800 weight-loss centers worldwide, clients who enroll in our program choose from a wide variety of highly flavored and textured breakfast, lunch, and dinner entrees, as well as desserts, beverages, and snacks. The snacks are specially formulated to be high in flavor and texture to satisfy those between-meal cravings that cause many overweight people to drop off a weight-control program. All Nutri/System food is *real food*—easy to prepare, and calorie- and portion-controlled. And our meal plan is carefully structured so clients get the nutritional balance they need each day.

Just as important, our clients visit our centers weekly for one-on-one nutritional guidance and counseling, as well as group behavior classes in which they learn how to change those habits that have contributed to their weight. And clients who purchase the Full Service or Premier Program also receive an exclusive, self-paced activity plan to help them make a gradual transition to a more active lifestyle. Finally, there's a one-year Maintenance Program to help Full Service and Premier Program clients control their weight once they've lost it.

The Nutri/System Weight-Loss Cookbook

With *The Nutri/System Flavor Set-Point Weight-Loss Cookbook,* we are introducing to the public for the first time the concept of heightened flavor and texture in recipes you can cook at home, all without adding excessive calories, fat, or salt. Here you will find hundreds of specially created recipes that are nutritionally sound, but still rich in all the tastes and textures usually found only in high-fat, high-calorie foods. These flavorful recipes embody all the tested weight-loss principles underlying the Nutri/System Weight Loss Meal Plan's success.

From our years of experience, we know how easy it is for dieters to deviate from their weight-loss commitment. How hard it is to plan and cook well-balanced meals. How tempting it is for cooks to nibble when they're around food. How frustrating it is to cook for the family

—then sit down to a plate of lettuce and cottage cheese. We have designed *The Nutri/System Flavor Set-Point Weight-Loss Cookbook* to make it easy for people like you to master weight-control cooking. Each recipe lists its caloric and nutritional content, as well as its food exchange values, according to the principles established by the American Diabetic Association and the American Dietetic Association.

You'll also find many suggestions for using these recipes in a weight-control program that appeals to your own needs. There are fourteen days of menus, and, depending on your own needs, you can choose among three menu plans—one for 1300 calories a day, another for 1500 calories a day, and a third for 2000 calories a day.

This weight-control book will also help you turn destructive eating patterns into productive weight management. For instance, you'll find tips to bolster your resolve under all kinds of circumstances—when you're the host or hostess, when you're a guest, when you travel, when you're at home, when you're alone, and when you're the one in a non-dieting household who has to prepare the food.

Perhaps most important, these are recipes that you can prepare and enjoy with your family and friends. Even the slimmest among them will find these nutritious, flavorful, and filling selections every bit as good as their everyday, high-calorie, high-sodium, high-fat favorites. You now have the freedom to share your new recipes with others—and they probably won't even know the difference. But you will.

We at Nutri/System, Inc., hope this book gives you a flavorful taste of the basics of the Nutri/System Weight Loss Meal Plan that has been successful for millions of people.

Stuart Shapiro, M.D., M.P.H.
SENIOR VICE PRESIDENT OF HEALTH AND SCIENTIFIC AFFAIRS
NATIONAL MEDICAL DIRECTOR
CHAIRMAN, NATIONAL HEALTH SCIENCES ADVISORY BOARD
NUTRI/SYSTEM, INC.

I. Weight Control the Nutri/System Way

The Nutri/System Meal Plan is well balanced and nutritious. It is designed to meet the U.S. Recommended Daily Allowances (U.S. RDA) as well as the dietary guidelines of leading health organizations. (This does not imply any endorsement by any particular health organization.)

The Flavor and Texture Set-Point Theory

A WEIGHT-CONTROL program doesn't have to take the fun out of food. That's one of the first things I assure my patients. There are ways to eat and to cook that will promote weight loss and help you control your weight, no matter how much you love to eat.

That's the challenge I believe I have solved with my Flavor and Texture Set-Point Theory. It's a delicious and healthy way to long-term weight control: low-fat, nutritious dishes full of intense tastes and textures, and delectable, zesty meals that let you feel satisfied with less food for healthy weight control. As long as you eat high-flavor and high-texture foods low in fat, you will never have to worry about your weight.

I came to this seemingly simple idea after listening to many patients in therapy over the nineteen years that I've been studying obesity. Nothing has taught me as much as the people I have treated for weight loss. Every time I ask them why they think they're overweight, most of them say, "Because I like the taste of food."

From my patients I've discovered that the main characteristic distinguishing overweight people from their leaner counterparts is simply that they want more intense and varied taste, aroma, and texture from their food. Unfortunately, those usually come in foods that contain high levels of fat. These people don't have an "overweight" personality, only a heightened sensory pleasure in eating. They have what I call an exaggerated flavor and texture "set point." They often say, "I'm not hungry, but I'm not satisfied." The most important thing for them to learn is to separate the idea of flavor from caloric density. Flavor is not fattening. Once you uncouple the con-

---

Alcohol and cigarettes drive up flavor set points by stimulating taste buds and odor receptors. People who quit drinking or smoking often turn to food for the flavor they're missing.

---

cept that tasty equals fattening, you can take pleasure in highly flavored foods — as long as they are also low in fat and calories.

Each of us, whether we're thin or overweight, has a set point for flavor and texture in food. We must derive a certain level of satisfaction from what we eat and drink before we feel sated. That level is our set point. And everyone's is different. Some people — usually thin ones — are satisfied with very little diversity in their meals; others — commonly overweight people — need many taste sensations. Why do some people overeat with an appetizer and a main dish, and still want dessert? They're looking for more taste and texture.

Because overweight people have accustomed themselves to an overabundance of taste, smell, and texture sensations, they have developed a need to eat that way. And since most conventional diets fail to provide enough flavor or texture, dieters are forced to seek them. When they binge on highly flavored foods, usually rich in fats and salt, they are likely to drive their flavor set point still higher.

Another cause for high set points is that overweight people tend to eat when they are bored or angry or frustrated. The simple act of eating more accustoms them to greater amounts of flavor during the course of a day. In fact, most Americans have high set points because, as a melting-pot culture, we are exposed to a wide variety of exotic foods — for example, Mexican, Cuban, Creole, Latin, Asian — with a wide range of textures and tastes.

Taste Is on Your Tongue

Taste is the sensation that occurs on your tongue when your taste buds are stimulated. Sweet, sour, salty, and bitter are the four "taste" words in the English language, but we actually experience many other tastes. For instance, you might describe the taste of hard water as alkaline, or the taste of cooked meat as "meaty."

The Perception in Your Nose

The yeasty aroma of bread baking. The spicy scent of an apple pie. The nutty odor of onions browning in butter. Just thinking about them makes the mouth water. The sense of smell, even more intensely than the sight of food, triggers the urge to eat.

It also stimulates our memories, as Marcel Proust wrote so evocatively in *Remembrance of Things Past*: ". . . the smell and taste of things remain poised a long time, like souls, ready to remind us. . . ." The taste of madeleines kindled Proust's memories, just as the aroma of roasting turkey and spicy pumpkin pie evokes family gatherings.

It is not necessarily that people who overeat have a better developed sense of smell than other people, but they pay more attention to food. In fact, they can identify more types of food with their eyes covered than other people can. In overweight people, a heightened sense of smell and taste is really learned, just as obesity is a learned behavior. Moreover, our vocabulary for describing smells is much richer than for taste; we often convert the name of the food itself to an adjective, as in minty, camphoraceous, fruity.

A lot of what you think is taste is actually smell. Smell is the stimulation of receptors in the nose. However, you receive most food aromas not through your nostrils, but through the back of your throat, by what is called retronasal olfaction.

Most odors are fat-soluble; smell molecules gravitate to the fat in food. For example, when you skim the fat off chicken soup, you are also removing 95 percent of the aroma. One of the reasons overweight people like food high in fat is because those foods have the most enticing aromas. The recipes we have developed are designed to retain the intense aroma that overweight people prefer by adding more flavor to low-fat foods.

Taste + Aroma = Flavor

How do we know how much flavor an overweight person wants during a day? To find out, I studied three groups of people—overweight dieters, overweight non-dieters, and some of ideal weight. I described twenty different common tastes, smells, and textures, and asked them how many bites of these different foods they needed during a day. Not surprisingly, those without weight problems needed the fewest, and overweight dieters craved the most — especially if those bites were sweet, chewy, crunchy, creamy, elastic, salty, or chocolate. The thinnest people had the shortest lists. The biggest surprise was the number of overweight people, whether they were dieting or not, who said there was really no limit to how much sweetness would satisfy them over a day; half of them said it would take a hundred bites or more. And most of their food preferences were high in fat, too.

Texture = "Mouth Feel" + Sound

Over the last twenty years, advertising has made us all texture-crazy. "Crunchy granola," "creamy gravy," "fruit-juicy gum" — the mouth-watering messages bombard us from all sides. They are the hardest to resist for people who want to lose weight. These people are acutely aware of texture, and the blander their food, the more they miss it.

How many food textures can you name? Crunchy, chewy, and creamy immediately come to mind. Most people name these and perhaps a couple of other favorites. But food comes in a wide range of textures, and I have found that overweight people have a great need for both variety and intensity of "mouth feels." I knew I was on to something when a patient of mine described what she most missed about giving up pizza: the pull of the cheese as she took the wedge out of her mouth after a bite. "That pull," she recalled wistfully. I realized it was the elasticity, a key sensory dimension, that was missing.

Texture is basically a combination of "mouth feel" plus the sound you get when you chew on foods. For example, both crispy and crunchy foods shatter in the mouth and promise fresh, appetizing, pleasant fare, but crispy (celery, potato chips) has a higher pitch than crunchy (nuts). You anticipate the texture of a dish at your first sight of it. If the way the food ultimately feels and sounds doesn't match your anticipatory vision, you won't enjoy it.

If you want to find out how important texture is to you, take this test. From the following list of food textures,[1] check how many you need during a three-day period in order to feel satisfied:

1. List of textural characteristics developed by Alina S. Szczesniak and Elaine Z. Skinner, researchers at General Foods Corp.

soft	firm	hard	crumbly	crunchy	slippery
crisp	chewy	tough	granular	tender	powdery
gummy	thick	wet	fibrous	sticky	brittle
thin	moist	dry	mealy	chalky	stringy
gooey	oily	flaky	watery	lumpy	rubbery
airy	greasy	tacky	fluffy	grainy	elastic
sandy	pulpy	pasty	creamy	springy	doughy
heavy	juicy	light	mushy	gritty	slimy
spongy	soggy	smooth			

I conducted a similar test at my laboratory with a group of overweight and a group of thin people. It was no surprise that the overweight people overwhelmingly checked more textures than the thin ones. They especially noted crumbly (as in cakes, cookies, crackers, and pie crust), brittle (nuts, potato chips, and bacon), gummy (taffy, caramel, pizza, and gum), gooey (peanut butter, syrup, fudge), oily (salad dressing, pizza), greasy (french fries, sausage), granular (sugar, cereal, rice, peas), creamy (cream, puddings, butter, and, of course, ice cream), and elastic (melted cheese). Incidentally, greasy, oily, and creamy textures are particular favorites because, in addition to their "mouth feel," they can deliver more aromatic sensations due to their molecular makeup.

Overweight people like to include many different textures in their foods, especially at dinner. Even a between-meal snack is likely to be both crunchy and chewy. When I ask some of my overweight patients to jot down the foods they wish they could eat and why, they often list six or seven textures per dish. Many yearn for a fast-food hamburger because it's crispy (lettuce, pickle), chewy, oily (salad dressing), greasy, juicy (tomato), granular (meat), and spongy. Or a chocolate-covered caramel candy bar because it is soft, gooey, tacky, sticky, chewy, and gummy. Other favorites are creamy pastas, buttered lobsters, barbecued ribs, pizzas, and chocolate ice cream.

On the other hand, when I put the same question to people without weight problems, they sometimes think of different foods

---

Puffy, aerated foods like puffed rice and puffed wheat have more texture and fewer calories than their denser non-airy counterparts, so a smaller portion will satisfy you.

> There are new ways to satisfy your cool and creamy frozen dessert longings: A ½-cup serving of American Glace, a fructose-sweetened relative of ice milk, has 50 calories and no fat or cholesterol. You can make your own frozen dessert quickly and easily in an anodized aluminum cylinder that you chill in your freezer, fill with non-fat yogurt or other mixture, and stir once or twice; Nikkal Industries' Donvier and Salton's Big Chill are two brand names. Non-fat yogurt has 45–75 calories and 0–9 fat calories per half-cup serving, in contrast to ice cream, with about 175–250 calories and 75–150 fat calories per half-cup serving.

and far fewer textures. They mention pears (firm, gritty), salad (crispy, crunchy, oily), veal marsala (chewy, tender, oily, fibrous), rice (granular, fluffy), and English muffins (crunchy, crisp, doughy, spongy).

Taste, smell, and texture are what attract people to food. If these didn't mean anything to you, you would have gotten thin long ago on lettuce leaves and cottage cheese. But I know they do matter, and I know you won't adhere to a low-fat diet unless it includes your taste, smell, and texture preferences. It is perfectly fine to say you eat because you like the taste of chocolate, or the creaminess of a cheesecake. It is only when you acknowledge your sensory preferences and pay attention to them that you will be able to choose low-fat foods that give you pleasure, and be able control your weight.

Why It All Works

The most important research that came out of my laboratory experiments is that people will be satisfied with a smaller amount of food as long as they get enough taste and texture. If you can include more flavor in a dish without adding more calories, particularly fat calories, you will eat less. This concept is one of the building blocks of the Nutri/System Meal Plan.

One psychological benefit of high-flavor foods is that they keep you from feeling deprived. Any diet that is going to work must provide a range of textures and flavors, or you will seek them in other, usually high-fat, foods. A flavorful diet prevents you from becoming what is called a "restrained" eater. These are dieters who hold back from eating many foods they love, but when they finally lose their restraint, they can't stop themselves from bingeing. One typical restrained eater tells me, "Every time I cheat, I might as well have some more cheesecake and a couple of nutty brownies. I've already done the damage." I remind her not to use the word "cheat"; dieting is not a moral issue but a nutritional one.

Another psychological boost comes from the fact that the high-flavor, low-fat way of controlling weight mimics normal eating patterns, so you don't feel out of sync with the world. Using the recipes in this book, you have the freedom to choose what to eat. You can have three meals a day. You can have snacks. Your meals are the same as everyone else's. Your family will be eating the same foods you are, so they will be eating healthier, too.

You can see why the Flavor and Texture Set-Point Theory is so important for your regular diet. When texture, taste, and aroma are intense and varied enough, overweight people enjoy healthy food, eat smaller quantities, and are better able to control their weight.

That's why the recipes we have developed are low in fat and high in flavor and nutrition; they have the taste, texture, and aroma you desire so you won't seek them from high-fat, high-calorie foods. They are scientifically designed to keep you from feeling deprived. What's more, when you combine your favorite recipes into three tasty meals, you can savor many of the flavors and textures you love in one day. (See Section IV for our suggested daily menu plans.)

Weight-Control Basics

WE often hear our bodies referred to as machines, and it's a good way to visualize the part that food plays in our lives and in controlling our weight. Food calories are the fuel that makes us run. Our bodies convert those calories into the energy we need to function. When we take in more calories than we can use at the time, we store most of them as fat for future use. As many of us have found to our dismay, sometimes there seems to be no end to the amount of fat we can store.

At its most basic, weight control is a simple equation: You maintain your weight when the energy you expend is about the same as the energy you take in; you gain weight when you chronically take in more energy by eating than you burn through exercise and general day-to-day activity; and you lose weight when you use more calories than you eat, forcing your body to utilize the energy it has stored as fat.

Now factor in some arithmetic: 3500 calories are stored in one pound of body weight. If in the course of a week, you take in 3500 fewer calories than you need to maintain your present weight — which forces your body to mobilize 3500 calories it has stored — ideally you would lose one pound that week. Just 500 calories fewer each day, and each seven days you should lose a pound of your body fat.

That's how weight loss would work if the body weren't a complicated mechanism. As you lose weight, however, your body adjusts to functioning on fewer calories, so eventually it doesn't need the fat reserve. This tends to occur most often on extremely low-calorie diets because you have lowered your metabolic rate and put your body into a starvation mode. Please remember: I don't recommend any sustained diet under 1000 calories a day. People on very-low-calorie diets—600 calories a day, for example—lower their metabolic rate and make it more difficult to keep weight off.

Right here I want to caution you not to try to lose more than two pounds a week, or more than 1 percent of your body weight. That slow and steady rate of weight loss is the best way to be successful. When you lose weight more quickly, you may lose muscle tissue as well as fat, and that ultimately defeats a successful diet.

Caveat Emptor

Beware of fad diets—the grapefruit diet, the water diet, the calories-don't-count diet, the lose-while-you-sleep diet, the drinking man's diet, the high-fat high-protein diet, the high-protein low-carbohydrate diet, the "place name" diets—because in the long run they don't work, and they can be dangerous to your health. There is only one way to lose weight—with low-fat, well-balanced meals, accompanied by behavior modification and regular exercise.

Over time quick weight-loss diets fail because they are not a viable way to control your weight. Weight control requires lifelong changes in food choices and in lifestyle. It's not over when you lose your excess twenty or thirty or fifty pounds; in fact, it's just the beginning. In this book you will learn why you need to change your cooking, eating, and exercise habits so you can live the life you want.

Your Weight Profile

One out of every four Americans weighs more than he or she should, and only half of these people are trying to lose weight. Here is how to tell if you are you among the overweight.

You can get a general idea of your ideal weight from the table on page 12, which was developed by Metropolitan Life Insurance Co. These ideal weights were revised upwards in 1983 after research showed that a few extra pounds were tolerable, but the National Institute of Health Consensus Development Conference on Obesity (1985) and the American Heart Association (1988) recommend the leaner 1959 standards.

A common rule of thumb is that you are considered overweight if you weigh more than 5 percent over your ideal weight, and obese at

1959 METROPOLITAN LIFE INSURANCE COMPANY TABLE
Weight in Pounds According to Frame (in Indoor Clothing).*

MEN: *Desirable Weights for Aged 25 and Over*

Height with Shoes 1-inch Heels Feet Inches		Small Frame	Medium Frame	Large Frame
5	2	112–120	118–129	126–141
5	3	115–123	121–133	129–144
5	4	118–126	124–136	132–148
5	5	121–129	127–139	135–152
5	6	124–133	130–143	138–156
5	7	128–137	134–147	142–161
5	8	132–141	138–152	147–166
5	9	136–145	142–156	151–170
5	10	140–150	146–160	155–174
5	11	144–154	150–165	159–179
6	0	148–158	154–170	164–184
6	1	152–162	158–175	168–189
6	2	156–167	162–180	173–194
6	3	160–171	167–185	178–199
6	4	164–175	172–190	182–204

WOMEN: *Desirable Weights for Aged 25 and Over*

Height with Shoes 2-inch Heels Feet Inches		Small Frame	Medium Frame	Large Frame
4	10	92–98	96–107	104–119
4	11	94–101	98–110	106–122
5	0	96–104	101–113	109–125
5	1	99–107	104–116	112–128
5	2	102–110	107–119	115–131
5	3	105–113	110–122	118–134
5	4	108–116	113–126	121–138
5	5	111–119	116–130	125–142
5	6	114–123	120–135	129–146
5	7	118–127	124–139	133–150
5	8	122–131	128–143	137–154
5	9	126–135	132–147	141–158
5	10	130–140	136–151	145–163
5	11	134–144	140–155	149–168
6	0	138–148	144–159	153–173

* For nude weight, deduct 5 to 7 lbs. (male) or 2 to 4 lbs. (female). Prepared by Metropolitan Life Insurance Company. Derived primarily from data of the Build and Blood Pressure Study, Society of Actuaries, 1959.

20 percent over it. But that doesn't account for our variety of builds, shapes, and body types. Take three people who are each 5 feet, 4 inches tall and weigh 130 pounds. The first is lean and large-boned, the second muscular, and the third has a small frame well padded with fat. Only the third would be called overweight. You can see from the table on page 12 that if you are 5 feet 5 inches and weigh

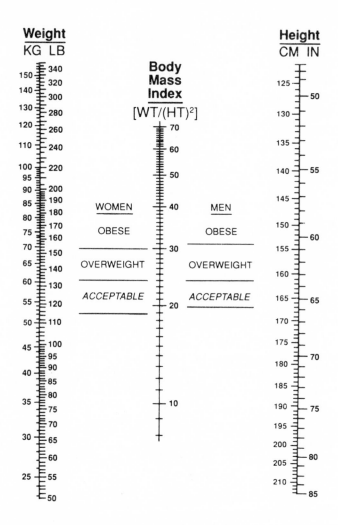

NOTE: Reprinted, by permission of the publisher, from G. A. Bray, 1978, Definitions, measurements and classification of the syndromes of obesity, <u>International Journal of Obesity</u> 2:99-112.

135 pounds, you are slightly overweight if you have a small frame, but not if you have a large frame.

If you are still not sure if you are too fat, take the pinch test. Hold one arm out and with your other hand grab the underarm flesh between the elbow and shoulder. If you are holding more than an inch of skin, you probably need to lose weight.

Another way of determining if you are overweight is to use the body mass index (BMI) to calculate the amount of fat your body contains. It is more accurate but a bit complicated because you have to convert your height into meters and your weight into kilograms (use the chart on page 13). The formula is to divide your weight by your height, squared (wt/ht^2). For example, I am 5 feet 3 inches (1.6 meters) and I weigh 125 pounds (57 kilograms). When you apply the formula (57 divided by 1.6×1.6, or 2.56), you will find my BMI is over 22. A BMI between 25 and 30 indicates overweight; greater than 30, obesity.

Born to Be Fat?

Whether you gauge your weight by the Metropolitan Life chart, the pinch test, or the BMI, one thing I know: Few of us on this earth were born to be fat. I am concerned that there is too much focus on the so-called genetic aspects of obesity. The bulk of scientific evidence shows that most obesity is not related to childhood but develops later. *Obesity is not genetic.* There may be a small genetic component that prevents some fortunate people from becoming overweight no matter what they eat, but most of us will gain weight on extra calories, especially excess fat calories.

Nobody has to live with being overweight. I am saddened by people who tell me, "It's in my genes. I'm helpless. I'll always be fat." I don't mind repeating once again that every one of us can lose weight if we do just five things: First, control our caloric intake. Second, cut

---

Women commonly store their body fat on their hips, thighs, and bottoms; men usually accumulate it on their abdomens.

> **Excess abdominal and upper-body fat puts people at greater risk for coronary heart disease.**

fats to about 25 percent—30 percent absolute maximum—of total daily intake. Third, raise the flavor levels of the food we eat so it is more satisfying. Fourth, change your eating behaviors. And finally, incorporate regular exercise into daily routines.

If you are overweight, you need to pay more attention to these factors. And if you have regained the weight you have lost, it is because you haven't changed your eating and exercise habits. Lifestyle, not genes, is the overriding cause of obesity.

Consider early man, who ate plants, fish, insects, and lean game that he had to chase (which provided his exercise). Studies show that his diet was only 21 percent fat, compared to the 40 percent or more that Westerners commonly consume. He did not eat cattle selectively bred for high-fat content and marbling, as we do, or high-fat cheeses, butter, and cream promoted by a strong dairy and meat industry, nor did he fry his roots in oils pressed from seeds. Our ancestors weren't overweight as are so many of us in Western countries.

Most people who eat a high-fat diet will struggle with weight. This is well illustrated by the migration studies of the Samoans, who got heavier as they moved from Western Samoa to American Samoa to Hawaii, and finally to San Francisco, eating an increasingly higher-fat diet that came with the domestication of animals for food.

Today people in oriental and third world cultures eat much as primitive man did—low-fat diets high in complex carbohydrates. And the few primitive hunter-gatherer populations that survive also have eating habits that closely resemble pre-agricultural humans. No matter what they eat, their fat intake does not exceed 25 percent of total calories. It is interesting that members of these primitive cultures who live beyond sixty years of age are free from the prevalent diseases

> **All fat is fat. Cellulite may look different, but it's still body fat with a new name and a dimpled look caused by poor muscle and skin tone.**

of contemporary Western cultures, including coronary heart disease, hypertension, diabetes, and some types of cancer. Historically, our bodies were designed for low-fat eating.

What Is Your Personal Calorie Quota?

Let's start with how many calories you need when you are resting. This is expressed as your basal metabolic rate (BMR), and it is influenced by many factors: It is higher if you are a man, and if you are overweight; it becomes lower as you age, and when you are sleeping. It fluctuates depending on how sedentary or active you are, and as you lose (and gain) weight.

Here is a rule of thumb to calculate your BMR, and the number of calories you need when you are resting: If you are a woman, multiply your actual weight in pounds by 11; if you are a man, multiply by 12.

Your BMR is, in effect, roughly equal to the number of calories you need to maintain your present weight *when you are at rest.* The more active you become, the more calories you need to maintain that weight. If you are moderately active, you will need more; if you are very active, you may need half again the number of calories. The more body fat you have, as opposed to lean muscle, the fewer calories you need to maintain your weight.

Once you have calculated your calorie base, you can figure out roughly how much less to eat in order to lose a pound or two a week. With 3500 calories per pound, cut your daily calorie base by 500 calories to lose about one pound every seven days.

Moreover, you can speed the weight loss process by increasing your activity, which burns more calories and forces you to use more of your fat reserves. Or, to put it another way, the more you exercise, the more you can eat without gaining weight. (To see how exercise translates into calories, see page 31.)

Only 100 extra calories a day from dietary fat can put on more than ten pounds each year.

Nutrition ABCs—A Primer for Healthy Weight Control

M OST people focus on calories as the key to losing weight. No question, calories do count—but the *kind* of calories you eat are every bit as important as their number. They should include all the nutrients essential for a well-balanced diet. When you are eating less, you have to be doubly sure you are getting all the essential food elements your body needs. Reduced calories, low fat, high nutrition, textural variety, and intensified flavor—that is the foundation of all the recipes we have developed.

Most of us know a lot more about good food than we do about good nutrition. To plan and cook healthy, well-balanced meals, it is helpful to understand what kind of fuel your body needs, how it is used, and where it comes from. Here is a primer of your body's basic nutritional needs. The recommendations are backed by the latest guidelines of the leading health organizations.

Please note: These guidelines are for people in good health. It is always wise to see your doctor before starting a weight-loss program, and it is essential for anyone with medical problems. Moreover, even healthy people should not eat fewer than 1000 calories a day without professional supervision.

Fat

As I have said before, excessive consumption of fatty foods has contributed to the prevalence of obesity. For Americans, it is important to reduce our daily intake of total fat, saturated fat, and cholesterol because high-fat diets cause obesity, and high blood cholesterol levels increase the risk of heart disease.

Fat is a concentrated energy source that has 9 calories per gram. We need a small amount of fat each day to absorb certain vitamins (A, D, E, and K), build cells, and keep the skin moist. However, the amount consumed by most Americans—37 percent of our calories, on average—is far too much. We can dramatically decrease our fat intake and reduce calories without sacrificing nutrients.

When you are counting calories, fat is a poor food choice because it has more than twice the number of calories per gram than carbohydrate or protein (each of which has 4 calories per gram). To put it another way, you can eat more than twice as much carbohydrate and protein for the same number of calories.

Fat is composed of several substances, but here we are primarily concerned with three of them—monounsaturated, polyunsaturated, and saturated fats. All three types have the same number of calories —about 120 in a tablespoon—but their differences are important

What foods to eat for their fat content

YES YES YES	NO NO NO
non-fat milk	cream, sour cream
non-fat yogurt	ice cream
buttermilk	butter, margarine
low-fat cottage cheese	most cheeses
egg whites	egg yolks, eggnog
breads and bagels	bread stuffing
tortillas	potato chips, corn chips
most cereals	most nuts, peanut butter
pastas and grains	mayonnaise
potatoes	most cold cuts
vegetables	chocolate
beans and peas	fried fish
fish and seafood	goose and duck
chicken (light meat)	most beef
turkey (light meat)	bacon, pork
chestnuts	sausages, frankfurters

because two promote health by reducing cholesterol and one presents serious hazards by fostering artery-clogging plaque.

Monounsaturated fats are good fats that reduce total serum cholesterol and may increase high-density lipoproteins (HDL) that cleanse the arteries by carrying away cholesterol. Good sources are olive oil and ocean fish like salmon.

Polyunsaturated fats, including corn oil, soybean oil, and other seed oils, reduce the level of serum cholesterol, but they also can reduce the desirable HDL.

Saturated fat is the culprit that increases serum cholesterol and risk for heart disease. Our bodies have no need for any saturated fat at all. Unfortunately, the foods most of us like best are laden with saturated fat — marbled beef, pork chops, butter, ice cream, most cheeses, and palm and coconut oils. Those tropical oils, which have been traditionally used in many commercial cookies and crackers, are actually higher in saturated fats than beef or lard. Major food companies are beginning to use healthier substitutes for tropical oils. You can see that saturated fats are the ones to cut back on to control your weight, lower cholesterol levels, and reduce the risk of heart disease. To help you choose appropriate low-fat foods, the nutrition information that accompanies each recipe lists saturated fat separately, and groups polyunsaturated and monounsaturated fats under unsaturated fats.

• **Limit the total amount of fat you eat to less than 30 percent of your daily calories — 25 percent or less is even better — and divide it equally among polyunsaturated fat, monounsaturated fat, and saturated fat. For a 1300-calorie-a-day diet, eat no more than 29 – 36 grams, or 260 – 325 calories; for a 1500-calorie-a-day diet, eat no more than 33 – 41 grams, or 300 – 375 calories; for a 2000-calorie-a-day diet, eat no more than 44 – 55 grams, or 400 – 500 calories.**

The saturated fat count in 4 ounces of a broiled fish like salmon is 1 – 2 grams; of a grilled skinless chicken breast is 2 – 3 grams; and of a grilled hamburger made with choice meat, 9 – 10.

Cholesterol

Cholesterol is a close associate of fat, but not a fat itself, and unlike some components in fat, it does not contribute to the texture of food.

Serum (blood) cholesterol is a soft, waxy substance in the bloodstream that is used to produce certain hormones and to build cell membranes and other cell components. It is carried in the bloodstream by lipoproteins. Low-density lipoproteins (LDL), popularly called "bad cholesterol," build up plaque on arterial walls, which can lead to cardiovascular disease. High-density lipoproteins (HDL), the "good cholesterol," help prevent heart disease by carrying the bad cholesterol away. Both are affected by the dietary cholesterol and the kinds and amounts of fats you eat.

Dietary cholesterol, as distinct from serum cholesterol, is found in animal-based foods. Egg yolks, whole milk dairy products, some seafood, liver, sweetbreads, kidneys, and other organ meats are rich in dietary cholesterol. Even if you didn't eat any cholesterol at all, you would still have a sufficient supply in your bloodstream because your liver manufactures enough cholesterol each day.

● **Keep dietary cholesterol to a maximum of 250–300 milligrams a day.**

Carbohydrates

Probably the best news that the weight-conscious public ever received is that pasta, rice, and potatoes — once perceived as the most fattening of foods — are now the fare of choice. These starches are

> **Saturated fat and cholesterol are not the same thing. Cholesterol is found only in animal products, saturated fat in animal products plus tropical oils, such as coconut and palm. In fact, many solid and "hydrogenated" shortenings, cocoa butter, and tropical oils are actually cholesterol-free, but very high in saturated fat that can elevate serum cholesterol levels.**

> **To minimize your risk of heart disease, your serum cholesterol count should be under 200, and the ratio between total cholesterol and HDL should be under 4.5.**

complex carbohydrates, not to be confused with simple carbohydrates, or sugars.

Complex carbohydrates are the more valuable kind. You find them in grains (breads, pasta, rice), beans, fruits, and vegetables. Foods rich in complex carbohydrates are dense in nutrients and have only 4 calories per gram. What's more, complex carbohydrates are not associated with any major disease.

Simple carbohydrates are sugars, both natural and refined. Fruits contain vitamins and fiber, and fructose, a natural sugar, which is regarded as less harmful than sucrose, a refined sugar that is used to sweeten most commercial candies and baked goods. Foods with refined sugar are high calorie and woefully short of nutrients, which is why we say they have "empty calories."

● **Make carbohydrates 55 percent or more of your total daily calories.**

Protein

Most of us grew up thinking protein should be the mainstay of our diets, so we are still apt to regard meat, cheese, and eggs as healthier than potatoes and pasta. That's why most of us still eat far more protein than we should, rarely realizing that protein-rich foods are almost always also high in saturated fat. Protein itself is low in calo-

> **For the same number of calories you can eat practically twice as much fruit, vegetables, pasta, bread, grains, cereals, and other complex carbohydrates as you can butter, cream, ice cream, cheeses, and other high-fat foods.**

> **Milk is an excellent source of protein as well as calcium (and other nutrients), but beware of the "low-fat" label; it means the milk is simply lower than high-fat milk. Better to choose 1 percent or skim dairy products.**

ries, with only 4 calories per gram; however, we must be careful that the protein we choose to eat is also low in fat. You do need protein to build and repair muscles, but your body requires much less protein than you may think.

 ● **Keep proteins to approximately 15–20 percent of your total daily calories. The National Research Council recommends about 44–63 grams, or approximately 176–252 calories, a day.**

Fiber

Fiber in the form of carrots and celery sticks has always been a diet staple, but lately we have come to appreciate it in many other foods. In addition to raw vegetables, fiber-rich foods include cooked kidney and lima beans, peas, spinach, prunes, unpeeled fruits like apples, whole grains, bran, seeds, and nuts.

There are two major kinds of fiber—insoluble fiber, which passes through the body intact, and soluble fiber, which disperses in water, forming a bulky gel.

Fiber, the structural part of plants, is essentially indigestible. This makes it excellent for controlling weight. First, its fibrous structure requires extended chewing, which helps satisfy the desire for texture. Second, its very mass makes you feel full and sated. Insoluble fiber increases intestinal regularity by adding bulk to foods as they pass through the gastrointestinal system.

> **High-fiber, high-texture foods like apples and carrots are excellent snacks because they require a lot of chewing.**

> **Eat whole fresh vegetables and fruit as often as you can. Squeezing the juice from fresh vegetables and fruits eliminates most of the fiber and some of the nutrients.**

Aside from its weight-control benefits, fiber seems to be helpful in reducing the risk of colon cancer and other intestinal disorders. There is also some evidence that the soluble fiber in certain foods, among them oat bran, helps lower blood cholesterol levels and may be helpful in preventing heart disease.

• **As recommended by the National Cancer Institute, include between 20 and 30 grams of fiber in your daily diet, together with a generous amount of low-calorie liquids.**

Sodium

Some people reach for the salt shaker even before they taste their food. Adding salt or sodium is such second nature that the average American consumes 4000 – 6000 milligrams of sodium a day. These levels are far beyond the 2400 mg found to be adequate and safe by the National Research Council. High levels of sodium are linked to hypertension (high blood pressure), heart disease, kidney disease, and stroke.

It is important to check food labels carefully, because canned and processed foods are major suppliers of sodium. Instead, use low-sodium and reduced-salt products that are available in a wide variety of products from canned soups, fruits, and vegetables to salt substitutes.

For dieters there is a benefit to limiting salt intake: Because salt retains body fluids, which will increase your weight, reducing salt will give you a clearer picture of your weight loss.

> **Salty foods can make you thirsty; avoid high-calorie drinks to quench your thirst.**

> Unsalted foods "salted to taste" average lower sodium levels than pre-salted foods, so prepare recipes with minimal or no salt, and adjust the seasoning at the table.

• Restrict your salt intake to less than 3000 milligrams a day; lower amounts are even better.

Calcium

Calcium is essential for maintaining healthy bones and, for young women especially, reducing the risk of osteoporosis. Because you will be cutting back on calcium-rich dairy products such as cheese and ice cream, turn to skim milk products, dark green vegetables, yogurt, and sardines.

• Current recommendations suggest you should try to get 800–1200 milligrams a day, which about 3 to 4 cups of skim milk or yogurt will provide.

Changing Your Eating Style and Behavior

WHILE eating a low-fat, high-flavor diet is crucial to losing weight and keeping it off, we must also attend to our eating behavior. Both are key components of the Nutri/System Weight Loss Program. Whether we realize it or not, each of us has a personal style of eating that we have developed over the years. It often comes from our early family life, and how we were taught to feel about food.

Did you come from a family who enjoyed eating meals and sitting around the table over food? Were there large portions and many courses? As a child were you urged to take second and third helpings? Or do you remember dinner as awkward and interminable, where you didn't feel part of the conversation? Did your mother insist you clean your plate? Was the radio or television set always on during dinner to catch the evening news? Did you have to be a fast eater to be sure of getting your share?

Some people eat standing up, out of carry-out containers or a pot, while others set a gracious table even if they're eating alone. Some people bring lunch to eat at their desks and others insist on going out. Some of us turn on the radio or TV as soon as we go into the kitchen, some of us like to read and talk on the phone when we are eating alone, and some of us enjoy a quiet meal.

All of us have feelings about food and eating that we learned early in life. Food symbolizes many things to different people — love, reward, solace, celebration, or a family bond.

Tips for Eating Healthy

Since all eating behaviors are learned, unhealthy habits can be unlearned and replaced with an eating style that will help you control your weight. Most important is to change the foods you select and the way you cook them. That means seeking low-fat products and ways to give them as much taste, texture, and aroma as possible, choosing new ingredients, and learning new ways of cooking. A Primer of Weight-Control Cooking (Section II) and the recipes (Section III) will help you cook and eat for a new thin lifestyle.

Here are some other suggestions that may be helpful—but, remember, they are not a substitute for low-fat foods cooked with flavor and texture.

- For three consecutive weekdays, write down *everything* you eat, including that taste of pie, spoonful of ice cream, extra pretzel. Also note the time, place, what you were doing, and how you felt. Do the same over a weekend. Now review your food diary to determine if you can find any pattern. This should give you some insight into your eating behavior. One patient of mine saw at once that she snacked only while watching television; she has solved this problem by keeping her hands busy doing needlepoint. Another discovered she ate all her high-fat food at her desk; she made a rule only to eat at a dining table. A third immediately realized that 4 P.M. was his difficult hour; now he schedules a short walk and a cup of decaffeinated tea or diet drink at that time.

- Eat only in places meant for eating—the kitchen, dining room, restaurant, company cafeteria. Eliminate such snack sites as your desk, den, living room, bedroom, car, movie theater, and on the run. You want to limit the number of places you associate with food.

- Make up individual plates of food in the kitchen so you can control portion size. If you set platters of food in the center of the table, you will be tempted to eat too many calories.

- When you are eating, concentrate on the food and its sensory properties. Enjoy the aroma, take small bites and chew them well, be aware of the taste and texture, and eat at a leisurely pace.

- Be alert for people who make it difficult for you to diet. Spouses, friends, and parents—the very people you are counting on most to

---

Twenty vegetables to snack on: artichokes, asparagus, bamboo shoots, beets, broccoli, cabbage, carrots, cauliflower, celery, cucumber, eggplant, endive, green beans, lettuce, mushrooms, peppers, radishes, spinach, summer squash, zucchini. Eat them raw or lightly steamed, with Fresh Herb Vinaigrette (page 122).

---

help you—may unwittingly undermine your efforts for varying reasons that are deeply embedded in the nature of their relationships with you. Among other reasons, a spouse may fear your new attractiveness threatens the marriage, friends may envy the success they couldn't achieve themselves, parents have been feeding you since you were born. It is important to be steadfast when someone suggests: "One little bite couldn't hurt." "I made it just for you." "It's a special occasion."

Make Every Bite Count

We have known for a long time that our senses play an important part in how we feel about food. The aroma of food, the way it looks on a plate, even its color all contribute to how food tastes to us—and that can have an important impact on dieting. There are many ways to utilize your senses to make dieting easier. Here are some strategies that will help you get more sensations from every bite—without adding a single calorie.

- Always put more than one kind of food on your plate. If you switch from food to food as you eat, never taking two consecutive bites of the same food, you will keep your taste buds satisfied and avoid what I call sensory fatigue. This happens because your taste and

---

Many people confuse hunger with thirst. If you think you are hungry, try sipping a glass of plain or carbonated water. This may satisfy you because you are really thirsty and not hungry.

> **You consume a lot of calories in liquid form — about 180 gallons of fluid a year if you're average. Limit them by changing to high-flavor, low-calorie decaffeinated drinks. Substitute whole fruit for fruit juices; 4 ounces of apple juice has the same 60 calories as 1 medium apple but none of the fiber or bulk.**

smell senses tire when they are overloaded with the same flavor, bite after bite.

You may already be familiar with other forms of sensory fatigue. Have you ever walked into a room filled with flowers and perceived a wonderful aroma, but after a short while, you don't detect it anymore?

- Avoid foods like sandwiches as the sole item on your diet plate. It is better to eat the components of a sandwich separately so you have diversity of taste and texture.

- When you chew your food well, you enjoy it more because, scientifically, chewing breaks down the food cells, releasing more molecules to stimulate your taste and smell senses. In addition, chewing sets up little currents of air in your mouth, wafting the pleasant aroma of the food up the back of your throat and into your nose, and increasing your sensory pleasure in what you are eating.

- Warm foods have a more pleasing aroma than cold foods, so you will be satisfied with less. On the other hand, you can sometimes acquire a taste for nutritious food you previously disliked, such as fish or cauliflower, by eating it cold because the odor is minimal.

- Warm foods take longer to eat than cold foods, often giving you the impression you have a bigger portion.

Exercise Is Important

EXERCISE is an essential component in a weight-loss regimen. In fact, it is one side of the equation: More activity, less food. They go hand in hand. You can't rely on exercise alone to slim down, and a diet without physical activity makes losing weight much more difficult. Both cutting calories in your diet and burning them through exercise is the most efficient way to reduce. When you diet without exercise, you can lose substantial amounts of lean tissue as well as fat; however, when you also exercise, you will lose more fat and less lean body mass.

Moreover, exercise not only burns energy while you are doing it, but it keeps your metabolic rate high for up to four hours after you have finished. That means you are still expending energy long after you have finished your workout. The habit of exercising regularly will help you maintain your weight loss.

Although practically all types of exercise improve your cardiovascular efficiency, they don't all have the same impact on weight loss. For example, walking at a brisk clip (4 miles per hour) appears to lead to more weight loss than swimming.

If you are not an athlete, don't feel you are about to start Olympic training. Workouts come in many forms, and if you garden, do yard work, clean your home vigorously, go dancing, or even run up and down stairs chasing children or carrying laundry, you are already burning up calories. The important thing is to keep moving, and to do it regularly.

Note: Be sure to visit your physician prior to beginning any exercise program, especially if you are over thirty-five or have not exercised regularly.

> This is how to monitor your pulse rate: Place two fingers high on your neck on one side of your throat, just under your jawbone, where you will be able to feel the pulsing of a carotid artery. Count your heartbeats for 15 seconds, then multiply that number by 4 to get your pulse rate, which is expressed as a count per minute.

How Much Is Enough?

Until recently, the minimum recommendation was to burn 600 calories a week, and you could do that in three brisk half-hour walks, or three 20-minute aerobic exercise sessions. That is a minimum. For optimal fitness and greatest protection against heart disease, my colleague on the Nutri/System National Health Sciences Advisory Board, Dr. Peter D. Wood, and his associates at Stanford University now recommend enough exercise to burn 2000 calories a week. That would be a daily 45-minute walk or a half hour of aerobic dancing every day. If you are overweight and not in shape, start slow and build up to the minimum. Later, when you have more stamina and confidence, you can consider Dr. Wood's level.

In any event, monitor your pulse rate five or ten minutes into any aerobic activity. Begin aerobic exercises moderately so your target pulse rate is never more than 60 percent of its maximum capacity. To figure your maximum capacity, subtract your age from the number 220; then multiply that by 60 percent to calculate moderate aerobic heart activity. For instance, if you are forty years old, your pulse rate probably should not exceed 108; if you are 55, you should keep it under 99. If your pulse beats faster than your target rate, slow down or take a rest. As you become more fit, you can increase your aerobic heart activity to 75 or even 85 percent of your maximum heart capacity.

> In addition to promoting weight loss, exercise lowers your risk of heart disease, slows osteoporosis, improves your cholesterol profile, and reduces tension.

ENERGY EXPENDITURE FOR 160-POUND PERSON

Activity	Calories Burned per Hour	Activity	Calories Burned per Hour
Aerobic Dancing	500	Running/Jogging (7.5 mph)	864
Badminton	308	Running/Jogging (10 mph)	1184
Baseball	308	Sailing	308
Basketball	556	Sawing Wood	556
Calisthenics	432	Shovelling	500
Canoeing	376	Skipping Rope	740
Carrying Load	500	Soccer	556
Cleaning Windows	308	Softball	308
Cross Country Skiing	616	Splitting Wood	500
Cycling (6 mph)	308	Square Dancing	432
Cycling (12 mph)	556	Squash	616
Cycling (18 mph)	992	Stair Climbing	616
Digging	376	Swimming (Low Speed)	308
Disco Dancing	308	Swimming (Medium Speed)	680
Downhill Skiing	432	Swimming (High Speed)	992
Golf	308	Table Tennis	308
Handball	616	Tennis (Singles)	500
Hiking	500	Tennis (Doubles)	308
Horseback Riding	432	Touch Football	556
Lawn Mowing	500	Volleyball	308
Racquetball	616	Walking (2½ mph)	308
Raking Leaves	308	Walking (3½ mph)	376
Roller Skating	432	Walking (4½ mph)	500
Rowing	432	Water Skiing	376
Running/Jogging (5 mph)	556	Weight Training	500

Tips for Timid Athletes

- If you are more than 25 or 30 pounds overweight and not used to physical exercise, start slowly with stretching and strengthening activities.

- If you know you won't consistently do strenuous exercises like aerobics and jogging, just take a plain brisk walk. In fact, walking is easier on your legs than jogging because there is less risk of knee and leg injuries.

Swimming, although fine for cardiovascular fitness, probably doesn't promote weight loss, according to the *American Journal of Sports Medicine*, because your body may try to maintain or even increase fat as an insulation.

Regular gentle exercise you can keep up is far better for you than intermittent workouts you won't realistically maintain.

- One good reason to exercise in the morning is that you will feel a sense of control that will help you stay on your diet the rest of the day.

- Include some exercise in your daily life: Walk up and down stairs instead of taking the elevator, park your car at the far end of the parking lot, walk to as many appointments as you can.

- Exercise with a friend; the buddy system is great for mutual encouragement.

Healthy Eating, Whatever Your Lifestyle

W HEN weight control becomes an integral part of your life— and it will—you will find you can adjust your diet to any situation. Life is full of family, friends, and fun that are associated with eating. You don't have to miss out on that when you make wise choices and plan ahead for good times. Here are some strategies that work in a world full of high-fat food.

Feeding a Non-dieting Household

No one likes to be the odd one out, and there is no reason why your family should not eat the same food you eat. Everyone can benefit from the same low-fat recipes. It is an act of love and kindness to your family to serve them the same healthy, flavorful foods that are good for you. What's more, if your children learn to develop taste preferences for low-fat foods, they won't have weight problems.

- Look at your new endeavor as an "adventure in good eating." Let your family know that your new lifestyle is important to you, and explain why you need their help. Tell them why you are going to prepare and serve certain foods, and that they may not be foods they are accustomed to, but that they are definitely not bland "diet" recipes.

- Look through the recipe index and begin your meal planning with selections similar to ones you currently serve and your family enjoys.

33

- Prepare meals with your children to teach them low-fat cooking and sound nutrition. Make meal planning and preparation an enjoyable family activity.

- Do the food marketing on your own, with a shopping list in hand. All too often spouses and children drift into the junk food aisles and drop in your cart just the kinds of foods you are trying to avoid.

- You have heard this tip many times before, but it bears repeating: Never, never, never shop for food when you are hungry.

- Clear your shelves of high-fat foods that are not part of your new lifestyle.

- When you are cooking one meal, use that kitchen time to prepare another dish or two for a future meal.

- Develop a repertoire of delicious low-fat desserts. You will find many of them in Section III.

- Try to make dinner time as democratic as possible. If you cook, let others clean up. If you clean up, avoid the leftovers.

- Encourage family members who must indulge in high-fat foods to eat them outside the house.

Solo Dining

The fact that it is just you for dinner should not change your new lifestyle. In fact, guard against treating yourself as a second-class diner. Pick a special meal from "Table for One" in the Menu Planner, Section IV.

- Sit down at an attractive place setting.
- Arrange your food attractively on the plate in moderate-sized portions.
- Don't read or watch television while eating, because you will be distracted from the sensory pleasures of your food.
- Treat yourself as well as you would treat any guest in your house. Bring out the good china and light the candles. You deserve it, don't you?

Eating in Restaurants

Finding low-fat food in a restaurant is sometimes difficult. It is also hard to select a low-fat option when your friends are enjoying high-fat foods that happen to have been former favorites of yours. At this point, however, it is more important to remember the consequences of high-fat eating. But take heart: Here are some ways to help you cope:

- Take the edge off your appetite with a light vegetable or fruit snack before leaving home.
- Don't wait at the bar. Nachos and peanuts are definitely hazardous, and alcohol is high in calories.
- Ask if you can be the first at your table to order. You won't be tempted by the choices of your dining companions.
- Choose fish or chicken, sauce on the side, and lots of vegetables without butter. Steamed and broiled—never fried—are the cooking methods of choice.
- Never—*never*—order a fixed-price meal. The temptation is strong to eat everything you are paying for.
- Try ordering two appetizers and no entree.
- If you drink alcohol, have only one glass. I enjoy seltzer with a twist or cranberry juice, a good substitute for the astringent taste of alcohol.
- Beware of the salad bar that offers potato salad, cole slaw, bean salad, sunflower seeds, croutons, and other high-calorie items, as well as a variety of creamy dressings.

Dry white wine has fewer calories than red wine, and wines in general have fewer calories than mixed cocktails and liqueurs. However, fortified wines such as sherry and port have a high sugar and alcohol content. To put drinking in caloric perspective, 3½ ounces of dry white wine have 80 calories, sweet wine, 102; 1½ ounces of 86-proof scotch, vodka, bourbon, rye, or Canadian have 107; and most liqueurs have about 75 calories an ounce. There are about 150 calories in 12 ounces of beer, and only 90 calories in light beer. Best bet: a dry white wine spritzer (2 ounces of wine with seltzer) at 40 calories.

When You Are Invited Out to Eat

Going to a friend's house for dinner can be troublesome because you are never in control. You don't select the food, the hour, or the format. When I am invited for dinner, I call my hostess and say, "I hope this doesn't interfere with your menu, but I only eat low-fat foods. I'm happy to bring something." A good friend will understand.

Here are some other tips to manage social gatherings:

- Before leaving home take the edge off your appetite with a low-fat snack, and, without being rude, arrive well into the cocktail hour.

- Eat half (or less) of what you are served, because portions will probably exceed your lifestyle limits.

- If the food is difficult to resist or extremely high fat, set aside a minimal portion to eat, then oversalt and pepper the rest so you won't be tempted by it.

- Politely refuse second helpings.

- At buffets, where there is usually a large amount of beautifully prepared food, take a few bites of many low-fat dishes. That way, you will enjoy many different tastes and textures.

- Use the smallest-sized plate. Even with a small amount of food, you are less likely to refill your plate if you are sitting with a group of people.

- At brunches high-cholesterol and high-carbohydrate foods of the sweet-tooth kind are definitely a problem. Have a small healthy breakfast at home, then stick to orange juice with club soda and spicy tomato juice, and hope there are English muffins, bagels, and fruit. Brunches are one place I remind myself: It's okay to leave this party hungry.

When You Entertain

Don't assume you are the only one who wants to eat low-fat food and that all your guests prefer high-fat dishes. These days, most Americans are concerned about their weight and cholesterol levels, but they do want foods that taste good. Now that you have changed your lifestyle and understand low-fat, high-flavor cooking, entertaining your friends is a wonderful way to introduce them to tasty new dishes they may never have had before. As you sample the recipes in this book, you will find a great many that are suitable for entertaining. When you serve your friends low-fat food, you are letting them know you care as much about their health as you do about your own.

You will find some party menus in Section IV with ideas for all kinds of festive gatherings, from brunches and picnics to dinners.

- Select simple, flavorful, low-fat dishes that can be dressed up with sprigs of fresh herbs, capers, slices of fruit, berries, and such.
- Use recipes you trust so you don't have to taste during cooking. Non-stick pans eliminate the need for butter.
- Serve dishes that discourage pre-party nibbling — a loaf of French bread, rather than rolls; a cake, rather than cookies; one large bowl of a dessert like a frozen soufflé instead of individual portions.

On the Job

An office setting has the advantage of keeping food relatively inaccessible.

- Whether it is lunch or a snack, never eat at your desk because your work will distract you from the calories you are consuming.
- Don't bring change for the food machines.
- Take a brisk walk away from your desk when the coffee cart with muffins and doughnuts rolls by. If you want something with your coffee, bring your own low-fat treat.
- Use part of your work break for a brisk walk, aerobic exercises, or just relaxation.
- Bring your own lunch. You will find suggestions in the Menu Planner, Section IV.

Traveling

Whether you are traveling on vacation or on business, chances are you will spend many hours at restaurants, with the opportunity to sample new dishes. There is no reason you can't do it if you make sensible choices. Remember, however, you will also find lots of pleasures on your travels that are not associated with food.

- If you are flying to your destination, investigate the airline's special meals. Ask about salad plates, seafood platters, and vegetarian meals, and order them on all connecting flights. You can also bring your own in-flight fare.

- When you are on the road, stock your car with canned tuna fish, chicken, oranges, and diet soda in case you can't find a suitable restaurant at meal time.

- Avoid hotel packages with three meals a day (American plan), no matter how reasonable the price; you will be faced with too much food.

- If you sample the regional specialties, make sensible trade-offs, choosing a light entree or skipping an appetizer, for instance.

- Think ahead about your vacation eating. For example, make a commitment to skip the snacks on a cruise, pass up rich desserts, or have only one glass of wine a day.

Self-Understanding and Weight Loss

I T is important to know what and how to eat for a new lifestyle, and to exercise. It is also useful to understand yourself and your behavior.

My colleague on the Nutri/System National Health Sciences Advisory Board, Dr. Michael Feuerstein, Director of Behavioral Medicine Programs at the University of Rochester School of Medicine, developed the Nutri/System Personalized Weight Loss Profile assessment that identifies the most common psychological situations that undermine successful weight loss. The complete assessment is available only to clients at a Nutri/System Weight Loss Center. The following highlights, however, will help you assess your own personality characteristics. Do any of these apply to you?

Job Stress: Do you think you have more work than you can handle? Do you do tasks your colleagues don't have to do? Work too many hours? Do you feel people are unfriendly or treat you unfairly? Dr. Feuerstein has found that the more stress people endure at work, the more likely they are to give up on a weight-loss program because it adds to their stress.

Social Unease: Are you nervous with people you don't know well? Ill-at-ease in unfamiliar social settings? Do you find it hard to walk up and join a group of strangers? If you are like most people who are uncomfortable socially, you have a hard time letting others know you prefer certain foods. You don't want to stand out, so you are more likely to eat and drink what everyone else is.

Self-consciousness about Being Overweight: Do you mind undressing in a gym or exercising with other people? Feel embarrassed when someone sees you eating a big meal? Hate to get weighed or see yourself undressed? If you answer *no* to most of these questions, you are not too concerned about the way you look, and that undermines a strong commitment to sustained weight loss.

Concern with Physical Appearance: Do you always make sure your hair looks right? Your hands are clean and your nails neatly manicured? Do you worry about blemishes on your skin? Are you aware of your best and worst features? Concerned about your posture? If you spend a great deal of time making sure you look as good as possible, you will be surprised to learn that you may be a diet dropout. That is because you probably have unrealistic expectations for how quickly and noticeably your appearance will improve.

Goal-Oriented: Are you hard-driving and competitive? Bossy and dominating? Need to be first and best? Do you usually operate in high gear, pressed for time, gulping your food, impatient if kept waiting? If you share many of these "Type A Behavior" characteristics, you are apt to be constantly disappointed in a slow and steady program — the safe way to lose weight — because your weight-loss timetable may be unrealistic.

Few Sources of Emotional Support: Think of your spouse, friends, neighbors, co-workers. Are most of them there when you need them? Can you confide in them? Do they boost your spirits when you feel low? How much do they really care about you? The more people you can count on for emotional support, the stronger your commitment and the better you will do on a weight-loss program.

Motivation to Diet: Do you want to wear more attractive clothes and look more attractive? Improve your health and reduce your risk of illness? Be more active and have a greater sense of accomplishment? Do you feel guilty or ashamed about your weight? Do you want to avoid criticism and feel better about yourself? The more times you nod your head as you consider each question, the more reasons you have for losing weight, the better you will do on a diet, and the more motivated you will be for the long haul.

Confidence in Ability to Lose Weight: Consider the number of pounds you expect to lose. Do you think you can do it? Do you *really* think you can do it? Just how confident are you — barely, moderately, extremely? The more confident you are in your ability to succeed and to last over the long stretch that weight loss requires, the better you will do on such a program.

Once you identify the factors that are likely to interfere with your best efforts, you will begin to understand what is holding you back. This is the first step to successful weight loss. In fact, in an extensive study at three Nutri/System Weight Loss Centers, the clients who charted their Personalized Weight Loss Profile assessments and, with the help of the Nutri/System staff, understood their problems, on average lost 24 pounds each after eleven weeks, while the dieters who didn't face their psychological difficulties lost only 12 pounds.

You can see how important self-awareness is to successful weight control. It helps you cultivate patience, a realistic view of how long the process takes, and, most of all, a strong commitment to lose weight. I see this happen all the time with Nutri/System clients and my own patients; they go on to lose their excess weight — and learn how to keep it off. You can do the very same, and in the process reap the benefits of good health, new energy, a sense of achievement, and a wonderful feeling of being in charge of yourself.

II. A Primer of Weight-Control Cooking

It All Starts with Food

IN low-fat cooking, every ingredient counts. If you plan meals around seasonal foods, it is easier to buy ingredients at the peak of their freshness. Shop at farmers' markets where the produce was probably picked that morning. Make a friend of your fishmonger, who will save the clearest-eyed fish for you, and your butcher, who will trim your meats carefully. And while you're at it, keep a few pots of fresh herbs on a sunny windowsill (try chives, basil, and rosemary) and an assortment of dried herbs in a cupboard, away from the sun. The more natural foods you cook yourself, and the fewer commercially prepared, packaged, and canned foods you eat, the healthier your diet.

When you buy ingredients, get only as much as you need for the recipe you're making. This is a lesson I learned from one of my patients who made a graham cracker pie crust for a wonderfully low-calorie pie — then ate all the leftover crumbs with a spoon. (It was the gummy texture she couldn't resist.) It would have been best for her to throw the remaining crumbs out.

Reading the Fine Print

When you buy any prepared foods, read the labels carefully. Watch especially for hidden fats, salt (sodium), and sweeteners under several names (see Sugar, page 57). Hidden fats include palm oil, coconut oil, hydrogenated vegetable oil, and lard, all of which have saturated fat and raise your cholesterol level. A common source of hidden fat is crackers.

Ingredients are listed in decreasing order of quantity, although

A "diet" food or drink may carry a lot of calories. "Low-calorie" foods may have too much saturated fat or salt. "All-natural" food may be full of all-natural saturated fat and refined sugar. "Enriched" food may be enriched with saturated fat. "All-vegetable" oils may be full of hydrogenated or tropical oils.

the precise amount of each item may not be given. Be sure that the ingredients you want in volume are named early, and those you want to avoid are at the end of the list, if they appear at all.

Remember that 1 gram of protein has 4 calories, 1 gram of carbohydrate has 4 calories, and 1 gram of fat has 9 calories.

Cooking Techniques

C ERTAIN cooking methods retain taste, texture, and nutrients far better than others, especially when you want to limit fat.

Steaming

You could hardly find a healthier way to cook food than to steam it. Preparing food this way retains all its natural vitamins and doesn't add a single calorie. Best candidates for steaming are vegetables and fish.

Steamers come in many shapes and sizes. One popular type is a simple round metal steamer made of perforated "petals" that expand and contract to fit into virtually any size pot. Three metal feet elevate the steamer above water level, and the pot's lid keeps the steam from escaping. There are also steamers available for microwave ovens.

The important thing about steaming is that the food is suspended over — never in — the simmering water. Set large pieces of vegetables, and fish steaks and fillets right on the steamer. Put small vegetables or anything with a sauce on a heat-proof serving platter first. You'll have tender moist fish and crisp bright vegetables.

When making soup stock, boiled meat, stews, or any other dish in which the fat cooks into the liquid, prepare the dish a few hours or a day ahead and refrigerate it; the fat will congeal and be easily removed.

Poaching

Don't confuse poaching with boiling—there's a world of difference between them. Boiling submerges food in rapidly moving water, which is fine for blanching or parboiling when the cooking time is brief, but which tends to leach out the nutrients, blanch out the color of vegetables, and make meat stringy when it cooks too long. Poaching, on the other hand, cooks such delicate foods as fish, vegetables, and fruit in barely simmering water that keeps them moist and tender, and retains the nutrients and texture.

Broiling and Grilling

These are excellent ways to cook beef steaks, several cuts of lamb, poultry, fish, some shellfish, and vegetables high in water content like eggplant. If you want to broil drier foods, marinate them first or coat them sparingly with corn oil or olive oil.

Successful broiling depends on intense heat, so preheat the broiler or grill for at least 15 minutes. Place all food on a rack rather than a flat pan so excess fat can drain off and the food doesn't sit in fat as it cooks. Use a cold grid for meats and poultry, and a preheated grid for fish.

Roasting

This dry-heat method of cooking is another way to extract fat from meats and poultry while bringing out their rich flavors. As with broiling, set all food on a rack rather than in a flat pan so excess fat drains off and the food doesn't sit in fat as it cooks.

Beef, lamb, pork, ham, and duck should be roasted without additional fat. Chicken and turkey should be lubricated with corn or olive oil, or lightly coated with a non-stick cooking spray, rather than basted with their own drippings. Low roasting temperatures (350°F.) extract more fat; higher temperatures seal in fat. Fish, shellfish, and vegetables like zucchini and eggplant roast beautifully, but may need a scant brushing of corn or olive oil to keep them moist.

Baking

Practically all kinds of baking sheets, pans, and tins are now available with non-stick coatings so breads, cakes, cookies, and muffins can be

---

When a recipe calls for browning meat, brown it briefly under the broiler instead of pan-frying.

---

baked in unbuttered pans. If you need to grease a pan, use a non-stick cooking spray like Pam, which has no cholesterol, no sodium, and 7 calories of fat (from corn oil) per 1¼-second spray.

Quick Sautéing

You can bring out the flavor of lean meats, poultry, vegetables, and fish by searing them at high temperature for a minute or two in a non-stick pan on top of the range. Many foods will require additional cooking at lower heat, but the initial searing locks in the natural juices.

Use liquid vegetable oils that are high in mono- or polyunsaturates to sauté lean meats, onions, rice for pilaf, and other sautéing you used to do with butter.

Stir-frying, a close relative to sautéing, uses just enough fat to lightly film the pan—with an unsaturated oil or non-stick cooking spray—and constant motion keeps the food from sticking.

Microwaving

Some foods were born to be microwaved, such as vegetables. You'll find that carrots, for example, taste almost like a different species. It's not just the speed of the cooking, but the way in which the microwaves penetrate and heat the food. And when food is covered tightly with plastic wrap, it creates its own cooking environment akin to steaming, and you don't need to add any fats or sauce.

Getting More Flavor without More Calories

Low-Calorie Tabletop Sweeteners

The best ones use NutraSweet®, a brand name for aspartame, offered to consumers under the product name Equal®. One packet has the sweetness equivalent of 2 teaspoons of sugar. Aspartame is such a good-tasting substitute that most people can't tell the difference between a food sweetened with it or with sugar. Approved since 1981 by the U.S. Food and Drug Administration, aspartame was shown to be safe in numerous scientific studies.

Salt Substitutes

Use these sparingly because all or part of the sodium has been replaced with potassium, and too much potassium may also be a hazard.

Fat Substitutes

Up until now, it has been almost impossible to make low-calorie foods that are as palatable as their high-calorie counterparts, especially the fried foods and creamy textures we love. Fat substitutes are being tested. All-natural butter-flavored products, which generally include a vegetable oil and some butter aroma, have no cholesterol, limited sodium, and only 4 calories in half a teaspoon. They are marketed as "sprinkles" under names such as American Home Foods' Butter Buds.

If you want to make a dish seem saltier, add lemon juice or hot pepper sauce.

> **Use fats and oils sparingly. You can almost always cut way back on the oils and fats in a recipe, and sometimes eliminate them altogether, without changing the taste. Rule No. 1: Always substitute polyunsaturated or monounsaturated oils for saturated oils and fats.**

Shake them on hot moist foods like baked potatoes, rice, noodles, and hot vegetables for a buttery taste.

Other fat substitutes are on their way to your grocery shelves. Simplesse is a low-calorie, cholesterol-free fat substitute made from milk and egg white proteins and marketed by The NutraSweet Company. Simplesse is currently available in Simplesse Pleasures frozen dairy dessert. It has approximately 1 – 2 calories per gram versus the 9 calories per gram in fat, and will be used in such creamy foods as ice creams and mayonnaise.

Another substitute fat is Procter & Gamble's Olestra, a no-calorie combination of sugar and edible oils that the body's digestive system can't absorb. If it is approved by the Food and Drug Administration, you will be able to use it for muffins, cookies, and deep-fried foods, including fat-free french fries. (Until then, try the Almost French-Fried Potatoes [page 224].)

Herbs and Spices

Nothing beats herbs and spices for no-calorie seasoning, especially when they are fresh. Chopped parsley, watercress leaves, and chives are common favorites. Here are other ways to spice up various foods.

artichokes	bay leaf, mint, savory, thyme
asparagus	marjoram, tarragon
beets	anise, bay leaf, caraway, coriander, dill, fennel, mustard seed, savory, tarragon, thyme
broccoli	oregano, tarragon
brussel sprouts	caraway, marjoram, sage
cabbage	caraway, dill, fennel, mint, mustard seed, savory, tarragon
carrots	allspice, anise, bay leaf, cinnamon, cloves, coriander, curry, fennel, ginger, dill, marjoram, mint, nutmeg, oregano, sage, thyme

cauliflower	caraway, curry, dill, tarragon
corn	chili powder, curry, oregano, sage
cucumber	dill, coriander, mint
eggplant	basil, garlic, marjoram, oregano, sage
green beans	basil, dill, marjoram, mint, nutmeg, oregano, savory, tarragon, thyme
lentils	rosemary, sage, savory, tarragon
mushrooms	chervil, garlic, oregano, paprika, rosemary, tarragon, thyme
onions	basil, caraway, oregano, sage, thyme
peas	allspice, curry, dill, marjoram, mint, oregano, rosemary, sage, savory
potatoes	bay leaf, caraway, dill, fennel, mint, mustard, oregano, paprika, rosemary, sage, thyme
rutabaga	basil
spinach	allspice, cloves, marjoram, nutmeg, rosemary, tarragon, thyme
squash	allspice, basil, cinnamon, cloves, fennel, nutmeg, rosemary, savory
sweet potatoes	cinnamon, cloves, ginger, nutmeg
tomatoes	basil, bay leaf, dill, garlic, marjoram, oregano, rosemary, sage, savory, thyme, tarragon
turnips	allspice, caraway
zucchini	curry, dill, marjoram, oregano
beef	allspice, chili powder, marjoram, oregano, savory, thyme
veal	chervil, mint, sage, savory, tarragon
lamb	cinnamon, curry, marjoram, mint, oregano, rosemary, sage, savory, sesame, thyme
ham	cinnamon, cloves
pork	caraway, coriander, ginger, marjoram, oregano, rosemary, sage, savory, thyme
poultry	basil, chervil, cinnamon, cloves, cumin, curry, dill, fennel, ginger, marjoram, mint, oregano, rosemary, savory, sage, sesame, tarragon, thyme

---

Marinate or heat herbs in oil to enhance their flavors.

> You can release more flavor from a lemon if you let it come to room temperature and roll it on the counter before cutting it.

fish, seafood	allspice, anise, basil, chervil, curry, dill, fennel, ginger, mint, mustard, sage, savory, sesame, sorrel, tarragon, thyme

Growing and Preserving Herbs

It's welcome news that no matter how ungreen our thumbs, no matter where we live, we can grow herbs easily. There are varieties for sun, for shade, and for almost any kind of garden soil. If all you can spare is a small spot by your kitchen door, fill a big basket with soil and plant a few of your favorite herbs. No outdoors at all? Line up pots of herbs on a sunny southern windowsill. Not enough sun? Use a grow light. Even when I don't get around to planting an extensive herb garden, I am never without pots of basil, tarragon, chives, and mint.

When the growing season is over, you can preserve your harvest by freezing or drying your herbs. I particularly like to freeze my excess bounty because frozen herbs taste almost fresh. For either process, wash the herbs and dry them well. To freeze, lay them in a single layer on a baking sheet in the freezer. After they are completely frozen, pack them into small freezer bags. Use them frozen in soups, stews, and hot dishes; defrost them for salads and cold foods.

You can dry herbs in an oven or, as I much prefer, in a microwave. For oven drying, scatter herbs on a baking sheet in a slow oven with the door open, watching carefully to be sure they don't get crisp. For microwaving, lay them on a sheet of paper toweling and cook for several minutes on high. In either case, store herbs in tightly stoppered jars out of the sunlight.

Some Food Facts

C ONTRARY to popular belief, **bananas** are not more fattening than other fruits. A medium banana has about 100 calories, the same as a large pear, and it is a good source of potassium, an essential nutrient.

The leanest cuts of **beef** are the eye round, top round, bottom round, chuck round, sirloin tip, flank, tenderloin, and lean stew meat. Avoid well-marbled (i.e., fatty) cuts. Don't buy ground beef; instead, trim the fat from a lean cut and grind the meat yourself.

About **butter, margarine,** and **oils:** Replacing butter with margarine will cut cholesterol but not calories; both have 36 per teaspoon. Margarine comes in different forms, some almost as saturated as butter. The softer the margarine, the more unsaturated it is. Choose tub margarines over sticks, and soft sticks over hard sticks. The first ingredient listed on the label should be "liquid," not "partially hydrogenated" oil. Look for a margarine that has three times as much polyunsaturated fats as saturated fats.

Margarine is a good substitute for butter in baking, but because it burns at a fairly low temperature, use vegetable oil instead for sautéing. For table use, you can save on calories with whipped margarine, in which the incorporated air replaces some of the solid fat, reducing calories by a third to a half. Or use butter-flavored sprinkles.

There are many kinds of oils, some of which are much healthier for you than others. They all have the same amount of total fat (about 4½ grams) and calories (about 40) in a teaspoon. They fall into these three categories:

Polyunsaturated oils: corn, cottonseed, safflower, soybean, and sunflower
Monounsaturated oils: canola (rapeseed), olive, peanut
Saturated oils: coconut, palm

You are likely to be satisfied with less oil if you use a highly flavored one such as olive, peanut, and sesame — but avoid saturated oils. (See Nutrition ABCs, page 17, for a fuller explanation of saturated fats and cholesterol.)

Cheese is a good source of calcium, but it is a prime offender for fat content. Cheddar, for instance, is 75 percent fat. Ounce for ounce, most cheeses have more saturated fat and calories than lean beef, lamb, and pork. Part-skim and low-fat cheeses will lower your fat intake, and that is why low-fat cottage and farmer cheese, and part-skim ricotta are diet regulars and the cheeses of choice in low-fat recipes. If you cook with other cheeses, use only a small amount for flavor.

Eggs have gotten considerable publicity lately for their high cholesterol content (over 250 milligrams in a "large" egg), but it is all packed into the yolk. Many recipes that call for whole eggs can be made just with the cholesterol-free whites, even such eggy treats as crepes. In general, add an extra white for every one or two yolks you remove, and be sure the dish is well flavored to compensate for the missing yolks. Frozen liquid egg replacement can be used in many recipes.

The nature of **flour** is determined by its milling process. Whole wheat flour uses almost the entire grain of wheat, including the nutrient-laden bran. Refined white flour discards the bran. Enriched white flour has some but not all of the original nutrients reincorporated in it, but none of the missing fiber. Graham flour is coarsely ground from the whole wheat.

Use vegetable oils instead of butter in such recipes as whipped potatoes, hot breads, pie crusts, and certain cakes.

Whole grain breads are more nutritious than those made with refined grains, even though those refined grains may be enriched. A slice of whole wheat or other whole grain bread has about the same number of calories as a slice of white bread the same size, but it has more nutrients, including fiber, especially if it is made from stone-ground flour. Toasting bread reduces its moisture, not its calories.

Fruit juice means the unsweetened juice of the fruit; fruit drinks, fruit punch, fruit ades, on the other hand, are made with water and usually a lot of sugar.

Whole **milk** has about 3.5 percent fat, low-fat milk has 1–2 percent fat, and skim milk is virtually fat-free. Other than their differing fat content, they are the same nutritionally and you can cook with them interchangeably. Buttermilk is made from low-fat or skim milk; it has a tart flavor and a thick texture.

The many shapes of **pasta** are generally made of semolina, ground from durum wheat. Pasta becomes more nutritious when high-protein soy flour or whole wheat flour are incorporated, or even when vegetable powders are added to produce green (spinach) or red (tomato) pasta — which doesn't alter the taste very much. Buy pastas made without eggs, but with enriched flour, because the B vitamins and iron improve nutrition. When cooked, enriched pasta has about 80 calories per half cup.

Popcorn is a good low-calorie snack — but only if you eat plain air-popped popcorn. Most popular brands for the microwave are loaded with fat and highly caloric, but one cup of fat-free popcorn has less than 25 calories.

Lean **pork** is getting easier to find. Least fatty are center-cut ham, loin chops, and pork tenderloin.

Poultry data: Chicken and turkey are the leanest. Goose and duck are fatty. Small birds are leaner than large ones. Dark meat has more fat and cholesterol than white meat. Much of the fat is in the skin, so remove it before cooking. When you buy ground turkey, it may contain some turkey skin; better to buy the turkey and grind the meat yourself.

Rice report: In terms of healthful nutrients, brown (whole grain) rice has the most, followed by parboiled or converted white rice, then polished white rice (by far the most popular kind), and instant rice, the least nutritious. The length of the grain affects consistency of the cooked dish, not the nutritional value. A ⅓ cup of cooked brown or white rice has 75 calories.

Salmon is a good source of monounsaturated fat, the good kind that helps cleanse the blood of artery-clogging cholesterol. Canned salmon is a great source of calcium, but note the sodium content on the label.

Sugar comes in many forms, all of them with 4 empty calories per gram and no significant nutrients. The common kinds are refined and brown, but sugars can masquerade under other names (many ending with "ose" and "tol"), as in dextrose, fructose, glucose, lactose, sucrose, maltose, mannitol, and sorbitol, as well as honey, molasses, maple syrup, and corn syrup. Some are sweeter than others; for example, the same amount of fructose (fruit sugar) is much sweeter than sucrose (common table sugar), so you need less. **Honey** is a mixture of several sugars, mainly fructose and glucose. **Molasses** is the residue left after sucrose crystals are spun off from sugar cane. **Brown sugar** is white sugar with the addition of different quantities of molasses to produce light or dark brown sugar. **Maple syrup** is the reduced sap of the maple tree. **Corn syrup** is derived from cornstarch. Each sweetener has a slightly different taste, but a sugar by any other name is still sugar. As you'll see on food labels, many processed foods contain several sugars.

Sweet potatoes have 25 percent more calories than white potatoes, but many people prefer their taste.

Veal is generally lean, but it has slightly more cholesterol than beef and pork.

Many flavored seltzers contain calorie-laden fructose and sucrose. Read the labels on carbonated drinks, especially those you think are low calorie.

When a recipe calls for:	Try:
Butter	Polyunsaturated margarine
Sour cream	Non-fat yogurt
Whole milk	Skim milk; buttermilk for baking
Whole egg	2 egg whites
Heavy cream	Evaporated skimmed milk
Regular yogurt	Non-fat yogurt

Unless **yogurt** is made with skimmed milk and is labeled "non-fat," it is made with at least some whole milk and can have a substantial number of calories. Fruited yogurt raises the caloric content even higher; a better alternative is to add fresh fruit to non-fat yogurt. Although commercial frozen yogurts and ice milks are laced with sugar, their fat content is much lower than ice cream.

Now that you know the basic principles of tasty, low-fat cooking, you will be able to translate your favorite recipes for your new thin lifestyle. Meanwhile, enjoy the following full-flavor, aromatic, high-texture recipes we have developed especially for you.

III. The Recipes

H ERE are almost 300 original high-flavor, high-texture, low-calorie, nutritionally sound recipes based on my research and my Flavor and Texture Set-Point Theory. They are crunchy, creamy, chewy, grainy, spicy, tangy, zesty — rich in all the tastes and textures people usually find only in high-fat, high-calorie foods. When you try them, you will see that they can satisfy your desire for flavor and texture, and they will keep you from eating too much.

Using these recipes, I have suggested two weeks of calorie-controlled menus, which you can find following the recipe pages. I have planned three groups of menus, each meeting different requirements for weight loss or weight maintenance. One set of daily meals is for 1300 calories, another for 1500 calories, and a third for 2000 calories; each includes a guideline for food exchanges. You will also find a helpful selection of recipes for entertaining, solo dining, lunches to take to work, and weekend picnicking.

To help you plan other daily menus, I have included caloric and nutritional information, as well as food exchanges, with every recipe.[1] (The reason that the total fat is more than the combined saturated and unsaturated fats is because it doesn't include other types of fats.)

When you start cooking, you will see that these recipes are deliberately sparing of salt and sugar, because we have used more nutritious ways to heighten flavor. I hope you will also discover many new tastes — curries, chilies, exotic spices, unfamiliar herbs — that are healthy, appetizing ways to add flavor and texture. Incidentally, it is

1. The nutritional data following each recipe comes from "The Food Processor II," a computer program developed by ESHA Research, Inc., in Salem, Oregon, and in most cases is rounded off to the nearest tenth. The food exchange values are based on the exchange system used by the American Diabetic Association.

no accident that you will find many foreign dishes. In countries of the world, such as Japan and Thailand, where the food is low in fat and cooks have learned to utilize their native spices and herbs for fuller flavor, there is very little obesity and heart disease.

A word about ingredients: We have taken special care to be precise about the amount and kind of every ingredient so every recipe is at its flavorful, nutritious peak. When a recipe calls for corn oil, for instance, please don't substitute olive or soybean oil, and never palm or coconut oil. Some recipes include wine and alcohol for flavor; if you prefer not to cook with alcoholic beverages, you can substitute alcohol-free wines, which are generally available at supermarkets. All the recipes have been carefully tested by a special panel of home cooks.

Most recipes list ingredients by their generic rather than their brand names. We tested the recipes with the following commonly available products. Their use doesn't constitute an endorsement, and failure to cite other brand names of similar products doesn't constitute disapproval.

Butter-flavored sprinkles:	Butter Buds
Frozen, liquid, cholesterol-free egg replacement:	Egg Beaters
Non-nutritive sweetener:	the aspartame product, Equal
Non-stick cooking spray:	Pam
Wheat and barley nugget cereal:	Grapenuts, NutriGrain
Reduced-calorie mayonnaise:	Hellman's

Since I love to cook as much as I love to eat, it is a great joy to share these special recipes with you, and to anticipate the pleasure you will have from sharing them with people you love.

Appetizers and Hors d'Oeuvres

Artichokes with Tarragon
Mustard Sauce
Broiled Mushrooms with
Crabmeat
Steamed Spinach Dumplings
Spinach Phyllo Bites
Crustless Spinach Mushroom
Quiche
Vegetable Terrine
Vegetarian Spring Rolls with
Hot and Spicy Dipping Sauce
Chili Rellenos
White Pizza with Broccoli and
Anchovies
Pepperoni Pizza with
Cornmeal Crust

Mexican Pizza
Smoked Turkey Bites
Spicy Cocktail Balls
Rye Squares with Crabmeat
Avocado
Clams with Garlic, Chilies,
and Fresh Basil
Futomaki
Hot and Spicy Nachos
California Nori Rolls
Beef Teriyaki
Parmesan Popcorn
Sweet Potato Chips

Artichokes with Tarragon Mustard Sauce

Fresh artichokes to dip into a mild lemony sauce that tastes like a creamy Hollandaise.

4 medium globe artichokes, about 8 ounces each	2 tablespoons lemon juice
1 tablespoon vinegar	⅛ teaspoon salt
	¼ teaspoon freshly ground pepper
Sauce:	½ teaspoon chopped fresh tarragon
¼ cup frozen, liquid, cholesterol-free egg replacement, defrosted	½ teaspoon prepared stone-ground mustard
¼ cup reduced-fat sour cream	

1. To cook artichokes on top of stove, bring a large pot of water to a boil. Add the artichokes and vinegar and return to a boil, then reduce to a simmer. Cook, uncovered, for 40 minutes. The artichokes are tender when an outer leaf pulls off easily. Drain and cool.

To cook in a microwave, place artichokes in a microwave-safe bowl, add the vinegar and ¼ cup of water. Cover tightly with plastic wrap, and cook on high for 12–14 minutes. Drain and cool.

2. Combine sauce ingredients and mix well with a whisk.

3. Cut cooled artichokes in half, and remove choke. Serve flat-side down with a dollop of sauce.

Yield: Serves 8 (½ artichoke per serving)

Each serving has approximately 43 calories, 2 g. protein, 2.1 g. total fat (0.7 g. unsaturated fat, 0.2 g. saturated fat), 4.2 g. carbohydrates, 0.1 mg. cholesterol, 2.4 g. fiber, 79 mg. sodium, 19.2 mg. calcium. Exchanges per serving: ⅓ fat, 1 vegetable.

Broiled Mushrooms with Crabmeat

Spicy, creamy crabmeat in chewy mushroom caps.

12 large mushrooms (about 1 pound), individually towel-dried

½ pound fresh or pasteurized crabmeat

1 tablespoon reduced-calorie mayonnaise

1 tablespoon plain non-fat yogurt

½ teaspoon crab seasoning

1. Preheat broiler.
2. Remove stems from the mushrooms. Save for a stock pot or discard.
3. Combine the crabmeat, mayonnaise, yogurt, and crab seasoning, and stuff into the mushroom caps.
4. Broil the stuffed mushrooms for 5 minutes. Transfer to a heated serving dish and serve at once.

Yield: Makes 12 large mushrooms

Each mushroom has approximately 27 calories, 4 g. protein, 0.7 g. total fat (0.5 g. unsaturated fat, 0.1 g. saturated fat), 1.6 g. carbohydrates, 15.5 mg. cholesterol, 0.5 g. fiber, 51.7 mg. sodium, 19 mg. calcium.

Exchanges per serving: ½ meat protein.

Steamed Spinach Dumplings

Chewy, slightly spicy spinach and turkey filling encased in moist dough. Serve them with Lemon Sauce (page 137).

5 ounces fresh spinach, washed and stems removed, or frozen spinach, defrosted

2 medium scallions

1 garlic clove

1 teaspoon chopped fresh ginger

1 tablespoon soy sauce

1 teaspoon grated lemon peel

½ pound ground turkey

25 round dumpling or square wonton wrappers

1. In a small saucepan, cook the spinach, covered, for 2–3 minutes over high heat, or microwave, tightly covered, on high for 2 minutes.

Drain well through a colander, then squeeze out extra moisture.

2. In a food processor chop the spinach with scallions, garlic, ginger, soy sauce, and lemon peel. Add the ground turkey, and puree for 10 seconds, until well combined.

3. Roll 1 tablespoon of this mixture into a ball to form the filling for one dumpling. Repeat this until you have 25 balls of filling.

4. In a wok or the bottom of a steamer pot, bring 3 cups of water to a boil. Set the bamboo or metal steamer in place, making sure the steamer basket doesn't touch the water.

5. If you are using round dumpling wrappers, place a ball of filling in the center of each, and gently bring opposite edges of the wrapper together, forming a half moon or crescent-shape dumpling. If the edges don't stick together, moisten your fingers with water and press dumplings at edges.

If you are using square wrappers, place the filling ½ inch in from one corner of the square. Fold the opposite corner over the filling to form a triangle. Moisten edges lightly with water and press to stick them together. If the wonton wrapper wasn't exactly square, cut off excess to trim triangle.

6. Cook the dumplings in two batches. Steam them for 8 minutes, or until they are firm to the touch. Remove the first batch of dumplings from the steamer and cover with foil or plastic to keep warm while you cook the rest, then serve immediately because they will begin to dry out and stick to the plate. To reheat dumplings, steam them again for 1 minute, or heat them in a microwave, covered, on high for 1 minute.

Yield: Makes 25 dumplings

Each dumpling has approximately 26 calories, 2.5 g. protein, 1.1 g. total fat (0.7 g. unsaturated fat, 0.4 g. saturated fat), 1.5 g. carbohydrates, 8 mg. cholesterol, 0.2 g. fiber, 42 mg. sodium, 9 mg. calcium. Exchanges per serving: ⅓ meat, 1/16 starch, ⅕ vegetable.

Spinach Phyllo Bites

This is a mini-calorie, open-faced adaptation of the delicious Greek dish, spanakopita. Packages of phyllo dough (sometimes spelled fillo or filo) are usually available frozen in supermarkets, but since it's easier to work with fresh than frozen sheets, try to get fresh phyllo at gourmet or Middle Eastern shops.

5   ounces fresh spinach, washed
    and stems removed, or frozen
    spinach, defrosted
2   phyllo sheets, each approxi-
    mately 12 × 17 inches

2   teaspoons melted margarine
2   ounces grated part-skim
    mozzarella cheese

1. Preheat oven to 450° F and lightly coat an 8 × 12-inch or 10 × 15-inch baking pan with non-stick cooking spray.

2. Cook fresh spinach in a sauté pan or steam for 4 minutes, or cook in a microwave on high for 3 minutes, covered. Drain fresh or defrosted spinach, squeeze dry in your hands, and chop finely. Set aside.

3. Meanwhile, melt the margarine.

4. Lay two phyllo sheets horizontally on a cutting board, one on top of the other. Lightly brush the right half with a little of the melted margarine, and fold it over the left half to form a rectangle roughly 12 × 8 inches. Carefully transfer the phyllo sheets to the prepared pan, turn the rough phyllo edges up ½ inch on three sides (the folded side will be smooth), and lightly brush the top of the phyllo with the remaining margarine.

5. Mix the spinach and cheese together, and spread over the phyllo.

6. Bake for 10 minutes, until the cheese melts and the phyllo dough browns. Cut into 18 pieces, and serve hot.

Yield: Makes 18 pieces

Each piece has approximately 17 calories, 1.1 g. protein, 1 g. total fat (0.5 g. unsaturated fat, 0.4 g. saturated fat), 1.2 g. carbohydrates, 1.2 mg. cholesterol, 0.3 g. fiber, 31 mg. sodium, 28 mg. calcium. Exchanges per serving: ¼ fat, ⅛ meat.

Crustless Spinach Mushroom Quiche

Tarragon-flavored vegetables in a light "eggy" base.

6 ounces mushrooms, sliced	½ cup grated Parmesan cheese
10 ounces fresh spinach, washed and stems removed, or frozen spinach, defrosted	½ cup skim milk
	1 teaspoon fresh tarragon or ½ teaspoon dried
2 eggs	½ teaspoon freshly ground black pepper
1 carton (8-ounce) frozen, liquid, cholesterol-free egg replacement, defrosted	¼ teaspoon salt

1. Preheat oven to 375° F. Lightly coat an 8-inch pie pan with non-stick cooking spray.

2. In a 3-quart saucepan cook the mushrooms and spinach until wilted, about 4 to 5 minutes. Drain mushrooms in a colander, and squeeze spinach to remove excess moisture. Chop spinach lightly, and set mushrooms and spinach aside.

3. In a medium-sized bowl whisk together the eggs and defrosted egg replacement, then stir in the grated cheese, milk, tarragon, pepper, and salt. Add the mushrooms and spinach, and mix well.

4. Pour the egg-vegetable mixture into the pie pan, and bake for 30 minutes on middle oven shelf. Let cool for 10 minutes to set before cutting. Cut into 16 wedges.

Yield: Makes 16 thin wedges

Each serving has approximately 55 calories, 4.7 g. protein, 3.3 g. total fat (1.9 g. unsaturated fat, 1.1 g. saturated fat), 2.2 g. carbohydrates, 29 mg. cholesterol, 0.8 g. fiber, 145 mg. sodium, 84 mg. calcium. Exchanges per serving: ⅔ meat, ½ vegetable.

Vegetable Terrine

This gorgeous terrine has crunch, color, and a different flavor in each layer. Make it for a party — it takes time, but it goes far, and you can prepare it a day ahead.

4 cups cauliflower florets	3 tablespoons butter-flavored
3⅓ cups skim milk	sprinkles
3 cups peeled and sliced carrots	2 packages unflavored gelatin
3 cups broccoli florets	

1. Lightly coat a 9×5-inch bread pan with non-stick cooking spray.

2. In a 2-quart saucepan cook the cauliflower in 2 cups of the milk over medium-low heat, partially covered, for 15 minutes, until very tender. Or cook the cauliflower and milk in a microwave-safe dish, covered, in a microwave on high for 10 minutes. Remove the cauliflower with a slotted spoon, put in a bowl with ⅛ cup of the milk it was cooked in, and set aside.

3. Using the same saucepan and the milk remaining in it from the cauliflower, cook the carrots over medium-low heat, partially covered, for 15 minutes, until very tender. Or cook them in a microwave-safe dish, covered, in a microwave on high for 10 minutes. Transfer the carrots to a bowl with ⅛ cup of the milk they were cooked in, and set aside.

4. Using the same saucepan, add broccoli and 1 cup of the remaining milk. Again, cook the broccoli over medium-low heat, partially covered, for 15 minutes, until very tender. Or cook in a microwave-safe dish, covered, in a microwave on high for 10 minutes. Transfer the broccoli and ⅛ cup of the milk it was cooked in to a bowl, and set aside.

5. Pour ⅓ cup of milk into a small saucepan or glass measuring cup. Sprinkle 2 packets gelatin on top. Let sit for 1 minute, then heat over low heat on the stove or 1 minute on high in the microwave until well dissolved. Set aside.

6. In a food processor, puree the carrots and their ⅛ cup of milk with 1 tablespoon of the butter-flavored sprinkles until smooth. Add 1½ tablespoons of the milk-gelatin mixture, and transfer the carrots to the bottom of the prepared pan. Spread evenly with a rubber spatula, and set aside.

7. Wash the food processor bowl, then puree the cauliflower and its ⅛ cup of milk with 1 tablespoon of the butter-flavored sprinkles until smooth. Stir in 1½ tablespoons of the milk-gelatin mixture. Carefully spread over the carrot layer. Smooth with a rubber spatula, and set aside.

8. Wash the food processor bowl, and puree the broccoli, its ⅛ cup of milk, the remaining 1 tablespoon of the butter-flavored sprinkles, and 1½ tablespoons of the gelatin-milk mixture. Spread over the cauliflower as the final layer. Cover the pan tightly with plastic wrap and refrigerate for 2 hours.

9. To unmold, cut around the edges of the pan with a knife. Place a plate upside down over the pan, then flip the pan and plate over. Let sit for 1 minute. The terrine will slide out easily.

Yield: Makes 8 ¾-inch slices as an appetizer, or serves 30–40 as a spread

Each serving has approximately 92 calories, 7.6 g. protein, 0.5 g. total fat (0.2 g. unsaturated fat, 0.2 g. saturated fat), 16 g. carbohydrates, 1.8 mg. cholesterol, 4 g. fiber, 289 mg. sodium, 173 mg. calcium.
Exchanges per serving: 3 vegetable, ⅕ milk.

Vegetarian Spring Rolls with Hot and Spicy Dipping Sauce

Chewy rolls filled with crisp vegetables to dip into a light spicy sauce.

2 ounces cellophane or rice noodles

1 slice fresh ginger, 2 × 1 inches, ¼ inch thick

¼ cup dry-roasted peanuts

½ fresh jalapeño chili pepper or ½ teaspoon crushed red pepper

3 small carrots, peeled and grated

2 cups fresh sprouts or 1 can (14-ounce) bean sprouts, drained

2 tablespoons low-sodium soy sauce

10 snow peas, trimmed, or ½ cup thinly sliced crosswise

2 tablespoons rice vinegar

10 egg roll wrappers

1 egg white, lightly beaten

1½ tablespoons toasted sesame oil

Sauce:

    1   teaspoon crushed red pepper
    ½   cup rice vinegar
    ¼   cup water
  4-6   packets of non-nutritive
        sweetener, to taste

1. Preheat oven to 400° F.
2. Soak the noodles in 4 cups of warm water for 10 minutes.
3. Finely chop the ginger, peanuts, and chili pepper in a food processor. Transfer to a 12-inch non-stick sauté pan.
4. Drain the noodles and add to the sauté pan. Add the carrots, bean sprouts, soy sauce, snow peas, and vinegar, and cook over medium heat for 3 minutes, stirring frequently. Remove the pan from the heat.
5. Lay an egg roll wrapper diagonally in front of you on the counter. Place ⅓ cup of filling on the lower half of the wrapper. Fold the bottom corner over the filling, then fold the right and left sides over. Roll the filled wrapper away from you, then place it on a foil-lined baking pan, seam side down. Repeat for the remaining egg rolls.
6. Brush the beaten egg white over both sides of each egg roll to seal the seams, then brush them lightly with oil. Bake for 15 – 18 minutes, or until crisp. Remove and cut each in half.
7. Meanwhile, combine all sauce ingredients in a small saucepan and heat for 2 minutes over medium heat. Strain the liquid over a serving bowl to remove the peppers, and serve with the warmed platter of spring rolls.

Yield: Makes 20 egg rolls
Each egg roll has approximately 53 calories, 1.9 g. protein, 1.9 g. total fat (1.6 g. unsaturated fat, 0.3 g. saturated fat), 7.5 g. carbohydrates, 2.5 mg. cholesterol, 0.9 g. fiber, 78 mg. sodium, 9 mg. calcium.
Exchanges per serving: ⅓ fat, ⅓ starch, ½ vegetable.

Chili Rellenos

A spicy appetizer with bites of firm vegetables and a hint of smoked cheese.

1   can (13-ounce) of whole pimientos (4 pimientos)
⅓ cup frozen corn kernels, defrosted
½ cup grated or finely chopped zucchini

1   ounce grated, smoked, part-skim mozzarella cheese
2   tablespoons finely chopped fresh cilantro
1   cup Spicy Salsa (page 129)

1. Preheat broiler.

2. Wash the pimientos carefully, drain in a colander, then wipe dry with a paper towel.

3. In a small bowl combine the corn, zucchini, smoked cheese, and cilantro. Fill each pimiento with ¼ cup of this "stuffing," then lay the pimientos on a baking pan. Broil the pimientos for 5–6 minutes, until the cheese melts.

4. Serve each pimiento on a small plate, with ¼ cup salsa drizzled on top and spread around it.

Yield: Serves 4

Each serving has approximately 81 calories, 4 g. protein, 3.3 g. total fat (2 g. unsaturated fat, 1.1 g. saturated fat), 11 g. carbohydrates, 3.7 mg. cholesterol, 4.3 g. fiber, 96 mg. sodium, 67 mg. calcium.
Exchanges per serving: ¼ meat, ¼ starch, 2 vegetable.

White Pizza with Broccoli and Anchovies

A crisp whole wheat crust with tender broccoli bits and salty anchovies under a chewy blanket of two cheeses.

Crust:

½ cup warm water
1 teaspoon sugar
1 tablespoon or 1 packet
   active dry yeast
1½ tablespoons olive oil
1 cup unbleached flour
¼ teaspoon salt
½–¾ cup whole wheat flour

Topping:

1 bunch broccoli (1¼ pounds
   with stems), stems removed,
   and florets coarsely chopped
1 can (1½-ounce) anchovies,
   including oil
3 ounces grated part-skim
   mozzarella cheese
2 ounces coarsely grated
   Parmesan cheese

1. Pour ½ cup of warm water into a bowl, add the sugar, and sprinkle the yeast on top. Cover and let rest for 5 minutes. The mixture will look tan and milky.

2. Add the olive oil and the unbleached flour, and stir until moistened but not lump-free. Cover and let rest for 10 minutes. The mixture will look bubbly and thick after 10 minutes.

3. Add the salt, then 2 tablespoons of the whole wheat flour, and stir until incorporated. Continue adding 2 tablespoons at a time of the whole wheat flour, stirring after each addition, until the dough is hard to move, sticks to the spoon, and pulls away from the sides of the bowl. You will need 6 to 8 tablespoons of flour.

4. Moisten your hands with a few drops of olive oil to facilitate kneading. Sprinkle about 2 tablespoons of the remaining whole wheat flour on a counter top or cutting board, and lightly roll the dough in the flour. Gently knead the dough by repeatedly pushing the dough down and away with your palms, then pulling it back toward you with your fingertips. Knead for 5 minutes. The dough should be slightly sticky at all times, but if it gets excessively sticky, incorporate the remaining flour, 1 tablespoon at a time.

5. Put this dough into a clean, lightly oiled bowl. Cover loosely and let rest for 45 minutes in a warm place.

6. Preheat oven to 450° F. Lightly coat a 10½ × 16-inch cookie sheet with non-stick cooking spray.

7. Steam the broccoli in a vegetable steamer until fork-tender, about 3 minutes, or microwave the broccoli with 1 tablespoon of water, covered, on high for 3 minutes.

8. In a 10-inch non-stick fry pan, heat 1 teaspoon of the anchovy oil, discarding the remaining oil. Add the anchovies and broccoli, and sauté for 2 minutes.

9. Lightly spread 1 tablespoon of whole wheat flour on a counter-top or cutting board to keep the dough from sticking. Roll the dough out into a 10½ × 16-inch rectangle. Place the pizza dough on the prepared pan. Scatter the broccoli and anchovies over the top, then sprinkle with cheese, and bake for 10 minutes.

10. To serve, cut the pizza in fourths down the long side and in fifths on the other side to get 20 pieces.

Yield: Makes a rectangular pizza yielding 20 pieces about 2½ by 3 inches

Each piece has approximately 78 calories, 4.5 g. protein, 3 g. total fat (1.7 g. unsaturated fat, 1.2 g. saturated fat), 8.6 g. carbohydrates, 6 mg. cholesterol, 1.4 g. fiber, 108 mg. sodium, 83 mg. calcium. Exchanges per serving: ½ meat, ½ starch, ¼ vegetable.

Pepperoni Pizza with Cornmeal Crust

An unusual cornmeal crust for a basil-flavored pepperoni favorite.

Crust:

- ½ cup warm water
- 1 tablespoon or 1 packet active dry yeast
- 1 teaspoon sugar
- 1 tablespoon olive oil
- ¾ cup unbleached flour
- ¼ teaspoon salt
- ½–¾ cup cornmeal

Topping:

- 1¾ cups crushed tomatoes
- 2 tablespoons tomato paste
- ¼ cup chopped fresh basil
- 2 garlic cloves, finely chopped
- 1 ounce 1-inch-diameter pepperoni, cut into very thin slices, then quartered
- 1 teaspoon garlic powder
- 4 ounces grated part-skim mozzarella cheese

1. Pour the warm water into a bowl. Sprinkle the yeast on top, and add the sugar. Cover and let rest for 5 minutes. The mixture will look tan and milky.

2. Add the olive oil and the unbleached flour, and stir until moistened but not lump-free. Cover and let rest for 10 minutes, when the mixture will look bubbly and thick.

3. Stir in the salt, then add ⅓ cup of the cornmeal. Stir until incorporated. The mixture will be hard to stir, stick to the spoon, and pull away from the sides of the bowl.

4. Lightly oil your hands with a drop or two of oil to keep your hands from getting sticky when kneading. Put about 2 tablespoons of the remaining cornmeal on a counter top or cutting board. Transfer the dough to the board, and lightly roll it in the cornmeal. Gently knead the dough for 5 minutes, pushing away with the palms of your hands, then pulling toward you with your fingertips. It should be slightly sticky at all times. If necessary, incorporate a little more of the remaining cornmeal into the dough, a tablespoon at a time, so the dough stays sticky without becoming heavy.

5. Put the dough in a clean, lightly oiled bowl. Cover and let rest for 45 minutes in a warm place.

6. Preheat oven to 450° F. Lightly coat a 10½ × 16-inch cookie sheet with non-stick cooking spray.

7. In a 1½-quart saucepan combine the tomatoes, tomato paste, basil, and garlic, and heat the sauce for 10 minutes over medium-low heat. Set aside.

8. Spread a tablespoon or two of the remaining cornmeal on a counter top or cutting board, or enough to keep the dough from sticking to the rolling pin. Roll the dough out into a 10½ × 16-inch rectangle, and carefully transfer it to the prepared pan.

9. Ladle the sauce over the dough, then distribute the pepperoni, garlic powder, and grated cheese, and bake for 10 minutes.

Yield: Makes a rectangular pizza yielding 20 pieces, each about 2½ × 3 inches

Each piece has approximately 66 calories, 3 g. protein, 2.4 g. total fat (1.3 g. unsaturated fat, 1 g. saturated fat), 3.5 g. carbohydrates, 3.5 mg. cholesterol, 0.8 g. fiber, 89 mg. sodium, 46 mg. calcium. Exchanges per serving: ⅕ fat, ½ meat, ½ starch, ⅕ vegetable.

Mexican Pizza

Think of these as crisp cheese wedges with smoked turkey, and you have the taste and texture.

1 7-inch flour tortilla (page 262)	1 tablespoon chopped scallion
1 ounce grated part-skim	(about ½ scallion)
mozzarella cheese	1 tablespoon chopped avocado
½ ounce smoked turkey, cut into	1 tablespoon Spicy Salsa
small strips	(page 129)
1 tablespoon cooked fresh or	
frozen corn kernels	

1. Preheat broiler.
2. Lay a flour tortilla on a baking sheet.
3. Sprinkle the tortilla with the cheese, the turkey, corn, and finally the scallions on top.
4. Broil for 1 minute, then transfer to a warmed serving plate. Top with avocado and salsa, and cut into 8 wedges.

Yield: Serves 8

Each serving has approximately 24 calories, 1.6 g. protein, 1.1 g. total fat (0.6 g. unsaturated fat, 0.5 g. saturated fat), 2.3 g. carbohydrates, 3 mg. cholesterol, 0.6 g. fiber, 35.8 mg. sodium, 29.1 mg. calcium. Exchanges per serving: ⅕ meat, ⅛ starch, ⅛ vegetable.

Smoked Turkey Bites

Cool juicy cucumber, potent horseradish, and smoky turkey in tiny triple-threat sandwiches.

¼ cup Horseradish Spread	1½ ounces thinly sliced smoked
(page 123)	turkey, cut into 1-inch squares
1 medium cucumber, sliced	
¼-inch thick	

1. Spread 1 teaspoon of horseradish spread on each cucumber slice and top with 1-inch piece of turkey.

Yield: Makes 12 pieces

Each serving has approximately 12.6 calories, 1.3 g. protein, 0.2 g. total fat (0 g. unsaturated fat, 0.1 g. saturated fat), 1.6 g. carbohydrates, 1.8 mg. cholesterol, 0.3 g. fiber, 34 mg. sodium, 23 mg. calcium.

Exchanges per serving: 0.

Spicy Cocktail Balls

Ginger, allspice, and mustard flavor lean turkey meatballs. Dip them in hot Chinese mustard or serve with Sweet and Sour Tomato Sauce (page 134).

¾	pound ground lean turkey	¼	teaspoon salt
2	egg whites	½	teaspoon dried mustard
⅓	cup fresh bread crumbs	¼	teaspoon allspice
2	cloves garlic, minced	2	tablespoons tomato paste
2	teaspoons minced fresh ginger		

1. Combine all the ingredients in a bowl. Roll into 1-inch balls.

2. In a microwave-safe dish cook in a microwave on high for 6 minutes, rotating the dish after 3 minutes. Or lightly coat a 10-inch non-stick fry pan with non-stick cooking spray, and heat it over medium heat. Add half the meatballs, cook for 1 minute, turn them over, and cook for 1 minute. Repeat for all raw sections, cooking for 1 minute each time until there are no raw spots, then cook for 1 more minute. Transfer to a warm serving dish and repeat with the remaining meatballs.

Yield: Makes 28 1-inch balls

Each meatball has approximately 32 calories, 3.4 g. protein, 1.5 g. total fat (1 g. unsaturated fat, 0.5 g. saturated fat), 1.2 g. carbohydrates, 9.4 mg. cholesterol, 0.1 g. fiber, 45 mg. sodium, 6 mg. calcium.

Exchanges per serving: ½ meat, ¼ vegetable.

Rye Squares with Crabmeat Avocado

Moist, chewy crabmeat spread on thin slices of dense, grainy bread.
Elegant.

4 thin slices good quality rye or pumpernickel	32 small watercress leaves or 1 small package of very fresh alfalfa sprouts
1 cup Crabmeat Avocado Dip (page 127)	

1. Cut each slice of bread into 8 1½-inch squares.
2. Spread ½ tablespoon of Crabmeat Avocado Dip on each piece.
3. Garnish each piece with 1 watercress leaf or a small pinch of alfalfa sprouts. Arrange the squares attractively on a serving platter.

Yield: Makes 32 1½-inch squares

Each square has approximately 17 calories, 1.1 g. protein, 0.6 g. total fat (0.5 g. unsaturated fat, 0.1 g. saturated fat), 1.8 g. carbohydrates, 3.7 mg. cholesterol, 0.5 g. fiber, 37 mg. sodium, 12 mg. calcium. Exchanges per serving: ¹⁄₁₀ fat, ⅛ meat, ¹⁄₁₆ starch.

Clams with Garlic, Chilies, and Fresh Basil

A spicy Thai appetizer.

24 small clams	½ cup Basic Fish Stock (page 100)
2 large garlic cloves, finely chopped	1½ tablespoons oyster sauce
2 hot jalapeño or cayenne chilies, finely chopped	1 tablespoon lime juice
½ tablespoon toasted sesame oil	½ cup packed basil leaves, finely chopped

1. Soak the clams in cold water twice to remove any dirt and sand, making sure each clam is clean and closed. If a clam is not closed, press it closed; if it stays open, throw it out.

2. In a 2- or 3-quart saucepan, sauté the garlic and chilies in the sesame oil for 1–2 minutes. Add the fish stock, oyster sauce, and lime juice, and bring to a simmer. Add the clams and basil. Cover the pot and let the clams steam for 5 minutes, until they open.

3. Put 6 clams in individual soup bowls or on small plates, and top with some of the remaining sauce, including the chilies and basil.

Yield: Serves 4

Each serving has approximately 98 calories, 12.3 g. protein, 2.7 g. total fat (1.7 g. unsaturated fat, 0.3 g. saturated fat), 6 g. carbohydrates, 31.5 mg. cholesterol, 0.5 g. fiber, 289 mg. sodium, 94 mg. calcium. Exchanges per serving: ¼ fat, 1⅓ meat, ½ vegetable.

Futomaki

A delectable Japanese delicacy — bites of chewy rice, salty caviar, and sweet eggy omelet strips rolled up in crisp and crackly nori seaweed. This is excellent with a hot, spicy sauce like Wasabi (page 131).

1 cup water	1 whole egg
3 teaspoons sugar	3 egg whites
½ tablespoon rice vinegar	4 sheets nori seaweed, each
½ cup sweet Japanese white rice	about 7 × 8 inches
(or any short-grain white rice)	4 teaspoons red caviar

1. Bring the water, 1 teaspoon of the sugar, and the rice vinegar to a boil. Add the rice, bring to a second boil, reduce to a low simmer, cover, and cook for 25 minutes. Remove from heat, and set the sweet rice aside.

2. Beat the whole egg, egg whites, and remaining 2 teaspoons of the sugar together with a fork, and set aside.

3. Lightly coat an 8-inch fry pan with non-stick cooking spray, and heat over medium. Add the eggs to the pan. As the eggs cook, lift the edges with a spatula to allow uncooked egg to seep underneath to form a flat omelet. Remove to a plate, cut the omelet into six strips (they will be different lengths), and set aside.

4. Holding one sheet of nori with one hand, carefully wave it over a gas flame or electric burner for about 10 seconds to toast slightly. The nori will change from a dark seaweed color to a brighter green. Set the nori aside and repeat for the remaining nori sheets.

5. Lay one sheet of nori vertically on a counter. Leaving a 1½-inch margin at the bottom of the nori, spread ⅓ cup of the rice evenly from side to side, and press the rice tightly into a compact cylinder across

the nori. Spread 1 teaspoon of caviar along the top of the rice. Lay one long omelet strip, or piece two shorter strips, over the caviar and rice, from one side of the nori sheet to the other.

6. Fold the bottom margin of the nori over the rice filling, and roll the nori up into a fat cylinder. Wet your hands, then press the loose edge of the nori roll to seal it. The sides remain open.

7. Repeat the procedure for filling the remaining sheets of nori.

8. Cut each roll into 6 pieces with a very sharp, straight-edge knife, cleaning it whenever it gets sticky.

Yield: Makes 24 pieces

Each piece has approximately 12 calories, 1 g. protein, 0.4 g. total fat (0.2 g. unsaturated fat, 0.1 g. saturated fat), 1.1 g. carbohydrates, 14 mg. cholesterol, 0 g. fiber, 22 mg. sodium, 4.3 mg. calcium.
Exchanges per serving: $1/10$ meat, $1/16$ starch.

Hot and Spicy Nachos

A favorite snack of crisp chips, hot pepper, and a light cheese melt, great with Spicy Salsa (page 129) or Green Tomatillo Sauce (page 130).

1 recipe Homemade Tortilla Chips (page 261)	1 fresh cayenne or jalapeño pepper, finely chopped
3 tablespoons grated part-skim mozzarella cheese (about 3/4 ounce)	

1. Preheat the oven to 400° F. or the broiler.

2. Place the tortilla chips on a cookie sheet. Sprinkle them with the grated cheese, and then the finely chopped hot pepper. Bake for 2 minutes or broil for 1 minute, until the cheese melts.

Yield: Serves 4

Each 10-piece serving has approximately 80 calories, 3.2 g. protein, 2.8 g. total fat (2 g. unsaturated fat, 0.7 g. saturated fat), 11.6 g. carbohydrates, 3 mg. cholesterol, 2.1 g. fiber, 30 mg. sodium, 70 mg. calcium.
Exchanges per serving: $1/3$ fat, $1/4$ meat, $2/3$ starch.

California Nori Rolls

With the Japanese genius for packing a lot into a small space, this traditional delicacy has cool cucumber, spicy ginger, creamy avocado, and chewy rice rolled up in crisp nori. An excellent accompaniment to these rolls is the condiment Wasabi (page 131). Nori seaweed and pickled ginger are available in oriental food stores or gourmet shops.

2 cups water	2 ounces peeled, ripe avocado, cut into strips
2 teaspoons sugar	
1 tablespoon rice vinegar	½ cup cucumber, cut into strips
1 cup sweet Japanese white rice (or any short-grain white rice)	1 × ¼ × ¼ inches
	2 tablespoons pickled ginger
4 sheets nori seaweed, each about 7 × 8 inches	

1. Bring the water, sugar, and rice vinegar to a boil. Add the rice, bring to a second boil, reduce to a low simmer, cover, and cook for 25 minutes. Remove from heat, and set the sweet rice aside.

2. Holding a sheet of nori with one hand, carefully wave it over a gas flame or electric burner for about 10 seconds to toast slightly. The nori will change from a dark seaweed color to a brighter green. Repeat for the remaining nori.

3. Lay the sheet of nori vertically on a counter. Leaving a 1½-inch margin at the bottom, spread ½ cup of the rice evenly from side to side, and press the rice tightly into a compact cylinder across the nori. Lay the avocado strips over the rice, then the cucumber strips, and finally press in pieces of pickled ginger along the width of the filling.

4. Fold the bottom margin of the nori over the filling, and roll the nori up into a fat cylinder. Wet your hands, then press the loose edge of the nori roll to seal it. The sides remain open.

5. Repeat the procedure for filling the remaining sheets of nori.

6. Cut each roll into 6 pieces with a very sharp, straight-edge knife, cleaning it whenever it gets sticky.

Yield: Makes 24 pieces

Each piece has approximately 34 calories, 0.6 g. protein, 0.4 g. total fat (0.3 g. unsaturated fat, 0.1 g. saturated fat), 7 g. carbohydrates, 0 mg. cholesterol, 0.4 g. fiber, 0.7 mg. sodium, 2.8 mg. calcium.
Exchanges per serving: ½ starch.

Beef Teriyaki

Slightly sweet, slightly salty, with the piquant flavor of ginger and tender beef strips.

1 **pound lean beef tenderloin, filet, or top round**

Marinade:

⅛ **cup low-sodium soy sauce**
½ **cup water**
1 **tablespoon ginger powder**

Sauce:

⅛ **cup low-sodium soy sauce**
2 **tablespoons sugar**
¼ **cup plus 2 tablespoons saki**

20 **4- to 5-inch skewers or long toothpicks**

1. Trim the meat of all visible fat, then cut it into pieces about 1 inch square and ¼ inch thick. There will be about 40 pieces.
2. Combine the marinade ingredients in a bowl. Add the meat and marinate for 1–2 hours in the refrigerator.
3. Preheat broiler. If using wooden skewers, soak them in water for a minute.
4. In a saucepan, combine the sauce ingredients. Bring to a simmer and cook, uncovered, over low heat for 8 minutes, or until volume reduces by one-quarter.
5. Thread two pieces of meat onto each skewer and discard the remaining marinade. Place the skewers on a broiler pan.
6. Brush the meat with the reduced sauce, and broil for 2 minutes, then turn the skewers over, brush with more sauce, and broil for 2 more minutes. Brush once again with the sauce and broil for 30 seconds. At this point the meat will be medium rare. Broil 1 more minute for medium, 2 more minutes for well-done meat. Remove the skewers from the oven and brush with the drippings from the broiler pan before serving.

Yield: Makes 20 skewers
Each skewer has approximately 55 calories, 7 g. protein, 2 g. total fat (1 g. unsaturated fat, 0.7 g. saturated fat), 1.3 g. carbohydrates, 20 mg. cholesterol, 0 g. fiber, 12 mg. sodium, 1.4 mg. calcium.
Exchanges per serving: 1 meat.

Parmesan Popcorn

The cheese gives this favorite snack a lightly salted flavor.

½ cup plain unflavored raw
   popping corn

¼ cup finely grated Parmesan
   cheese

1. Pop the popping corn in a hot-air popcorn machine according to manufacturer's instructions, or in a popcorn popper especially made for microwave ovens.

2. For microwave cooking, put a layer of popcorn in a microwave-safe bowl, sprinkle with Parmesan, and repeat in layers for the remaining popcorn and cheese. Cover with plastic wrap and microwave for 1 minute, until the cheese melts.

For oven baking, alternately layer the popcorn and cheese in the same way, and bake in a preheated 250° F. oven for 5 minutes to melt the cheese.

Yield: Makes 11 cups

Each cup has approximately 30 calories, 1 g. protein, 1.1 g. total fat (0.3 g. unsaturated fat, 0.1 g. saturated fat), 6 g. carbohydrates, 0 mg. cholesterol, 1.3 g. fiber, 0.6 mg. sodium, 1 mg. calcium.
Exchanges per serving: starch ⅓.

Sweet Potato Chips

Sweet and slightly crispy chips that don't need salt.

½ pound sweet potatoes
½ tablespoon corn oil

1. Preheat oven to 400° F. Lightly coat a baking sheet with non-stick cooking spray.

2. Slice the sweet potatoes by hand in very thin slices, or use a food processor with a 2-millimeter disk.

3. In a large bowl carefully toss the sweet potato slices by hand in the oil to coat the chips lightly. Lay the slices in a single layer in the prepared baking pan.

4. Bake the chips for 15 minutes. Turn each piece over with a metal spatula, and bake for 5 more minutes. Chips should be dry and slightly crisp. If not, bake up to 3 more minutes, checking every minute so the chips won't burn. Let cool for 5 minutes before serving.

Yield: Makes 8 servings, about 7 chips each

Each serving has approximately 37 calories, 0.5 g. protein, 0.9 g. total fat (0.7 g. unsaturated fat, 0.1 g. saturated fat), 6.9 g. carbohydrates, 0 mg. cholesterol, 0.9 g. fiber, 3 mg. sodium, 8 mg. calcium. Exchanges per serving: ½ starch.

Soups

Basic Chicken Stock
Chicken Rice Soup
Chicken Soup with Matzo Balls
Egg Drop Soup
Vegetable Barley Soup
Cabbage and Bean Soup
Six-Vegetable Chowder
Succotash Soup
Cream of Broccoli Soup
Creamy Orange Carrot Soup
Cream of Spinach Soup
Herbed Tomato Soup

Sweet Potato Soup
Pumpkin Soup
Beef Stock
French Onion Soup
Sweet and Sour Beef and
  Cabbage Soup
Basic Fish Stock
Fish Chowder
Tomato Clam Soup
Chilled Blueberry Soup
Cold Creamy Cucumber Soup

Basic Chicken Stock

A rich flavorful stock that's the basis of several of our soups, and is useful in many recipes. Use the cooked chicken in such recipes as Chicken Rice Soup (page 87), Fruited Curried Chicken Salad (page 108), Spicy Lemon Chicken Salad (page 107), and Chicken Fettuccine with Broccoli (page 167).

6	quarts water	3	small onions, with skins
1	4-pound frying chicken, including liver, neck, gizzard, or 4 pounds inexpensive chicken parts	3	celery stalks, including tops
		3	carrots, scrubbed
		1	teaspoon peppercorns

1. Combine all the ingredients in a stock pot. Bring water to a boil, then reduce heat and simmer, uncovered, for 1 hour, periodically skimming foam off the top as it rises.

2. After 1 hour remove the chicken and continue cooking the stock for 2 more hours.

3. Strain the stock through a colander into a large bowl to remove the vegetables. Let cool, then refrigerate. Fat will rise to the surface and coagulate for easy removal.

Yield: Makes about 4 quarts

Each cup has approximately 16 calories, 3.6 g. protein, 0 g. total fat (0 g. unsaturated fat, 0 g. saturated fat), 0 g. carbohydrates, 0 mg. cholesterol, 0 g. fiber, 50 mg. sodium, 0 mg. calcium.

Exchanges per cup: $\frac{1}{3}$ meat.

Chicken Rice Soup

Garlic, herbs, crisp vegetables, and grainy brown rice are the surprise ingredients.

2 garlic cloves, finely chopped	⅔ cup brown rice, rinsed
⅔ cup chopped onion (about 1 medium onion)	1 cup cooked bite-sized chicken chunks
8 cups Basic Chicken Stock (page 86)	1 teaspoon dried marjoram
3 celery stalks, cut in ½-inch slices	¾ teaspoon salt
3 carrots, peeled and cut ½-inch thick	½ teaspoon pepper

1. In a 4-quart soup pot, cook the garlic and onion in 2 tablespoons of the chicken stock until the onion is translucent. Add the celery, carrots, rice, and the remaining chicken stock. Simmer for 40 minutes, uncovered.

2. Add the cooked chicken pieces, marjoram, salt, and pepper. Simmer for 2–3 more minutes, and serve.

Yield: Makes 8 ¾-cup servings

Each serving has approximately 121 calories, 10.7 g. protein, 1.2 g. total fat (0.7 g. unsaturated fat, 0.3 g. saturated fat), 16.3 g. carbohydrates, 14.8 mg. cholesterol, 1.9 g. fiber, 288 mg. sodium, 26 mg. calcium.

Exchanges per serving: ½ meat, ¾ starch, 2 vegetable.

Chicken Soup with Matzo Balls

Light, spongy matzo balls and tender bites of chicken in a rich broth.

1 tablespoon oil	½ teaspoon salt
1 whole egg	¼ teaspoon freshly ground pepper to taste
1 egg white	1 cup cooked chicken meat
½ cup matzo meal	
¼ teaspoon salt	
7½ cups Basic Chicken Stock (page 86)	

1. Mix the oil, whole egg, and egg white together in a bowl. Stir in the matzo meal and ¼ teaspoon of salt, mixing until lump-free, then stir in 2 tablespoons of the chicken stock. Cover and refrigerate for 15 minutes.

2. In a 3-quart soup pot cook the remaining chicken stock with the ½ teaspoon of salt and pepper, uncovered, for 20 minutes, over medium-low heat to concentrate the flavor and reduce the volume slightly. Turn heat to very low while you make the matzo balls.

3. In a 3-quart pot bring 2 quarts of water to a boil. Remove the matzo ball mixture from the refrigerator. Lightly oil your hands, then divide the mixture into 12 pieces and roll into balls. They may look small, but they will puff up when cooked. Lower the matzo balls into the boiling water and cook for 25 minutes.

4. Remove the matzo balls with a slotted spoon, and add to the heated chicken stock, along with the cooked chicken meat. Cook for 2 more minutes to heat the chicken.

Yield: Makes 8 ¾-cup servings of soup, each with two matzo balls

Each serving has approximately 83 calories, 10.5 g. protein, 3.7 g. total fat (2.5 g. unsaturated fat, 0.8 g. saturated fat), 6 g. carbohydrates, 41 mg. cholesterol, 0 g. fiber, 276 mg. sodium, 7.6 mg. calcium. Exchanges per serving: ½ fat, ⅓ meat, ⅓ starch.

Egg Drop Soup

Light, sherry-flavored soup with the tang of scallion rounds.

6¼ cups Basic Chicken Stock (page 86)	¼ teaspoon salt
2 tablespoons low-sodium soy sauce	2 egg whites
2 tablespoons sherry	1 tablespoon cornstarch
⅛ teaspoon white pepper	1 tablespoon sesame oil
	2 scallions, thinly sliced

1. In a 2-quart soup pot, heat 6 cups of chicken broth to a simmer. Add the soy sauce, sherry, pepper, and salt.

2. Beat the egg whites lightly. Drizzle into the chicken broth mixture.

3. Mix cornstarch with the remaining ¼ cup cold chicken stock

until it is lump-free, then add to the soup. Stir until the soup thickens. Stir in the sesame oil.

4. Garnish with scallions, and serve.

Yield: Makes 8 ¾-cup servings
Each serving has approximately 31 calories, 1.12 g. protein, 1.8 g. total fat (1.4 g. unsaturated fat, 0.24 g. saturated fat), 1.6 g. carbohydrates, 0 mg. cholesterol, 0.06 g. fiber, 230 mg. sodium, 6 mg. calcium. Exchanges per serving: ⅓ fat, ¼ meat.

Vegetable Barley Soup

A colorful soup with the tender bite of crisp vegetables and the graininess of barley in a light garlic-laden tomato base.

1 medium onion, finely chopped	3 cups fresh spinach, packed, lightly chopped
4 garlic cloves, finely chopped	1 can (6-ounce) tomato paste
7 cups Basic Chicken Stock (page 86)	1 tablespoon chopped fresh thyme or 1 teaspoon dried
⅓ cup pearl barley	2 tablespoons chopped fresh dill
1 green pepper, finely chopped	
1 cup cauliflower florets	½ teaspoon black pepper
1½ cups diced zucchini	¾ teaspoon salt

1. In a large soup pot, cook the onion and garlic in 3 tablespoons of the chicken stock. When the onions are wilted, add the barley and the remaining stock. Cook together on low heat for 25 minutes, covered. Add the green pepper, cauliflower, zucchini, and spinach and cook for 20 more minutes.

2. Stir in the tomato paste, thyme, dill, pepper, and salt. Continue stirring until the tomato paste dissolves. Cook for 5 more minutes.

Yield: Makes 8 1-cup servings
Each serving has approximately 84 calories, 6.3 g. protein, 0.5 g. total fat (0.3 g. unsaturated fat, 0.1 g. saturated fat), 15.3 g. carbohydrates, 0 mg. cholesterol, 4.1 g. fiber, 278 mg. sodium, 55.3 mg. calcium. Exchanges per serving: ½ meat, ½ starch, 1 vegetable.

Cabbage and Bean Soup

Spicy, flavorful broth with crunchy and chewy vegetables.

1 cup dry white beans	½ head cabbage, shredded
3 cups water	¾ teaspoon salt
3 garlic cloves, finely chopped	1 teaspoon freshly ground black
¾ cup finely chopped onion	pepper
(1 medium)	2 tablespoons chopped fresh
3 medium carrots, peeled and	basil or 2 teaspoons dried
chopped	1 tablespoon chopped fresh
8 cups Basic Chicken Stock	thyme or 1 teaspoon dried
(page 86) or vegetable stock	2 tablespoons grated Parmesan
3 celery stalks, chopped	cheese
1 large zucchini, thinly sliced or	
cubed (1 pound)	

1. Pick out any pebbles and dirt in the beans, and soak them overnight in the water. Drain after soaking.

2. In a 3-quart soup pot cook the garlic, onion, and carrots in 2 tablespoons of the chicken stock for 3 minutes.

3. Add the celery, drained beans, and remaining chicken stock. Bring to a simmer, and cook over low heat for 30 minutes, uncovered.

4. Remove 1 cup of the soup, puree it in the blender, and pour it back into the pot to give the soup some "body."

5. Add the zucchini, cabbage, salt, pepper, basil, and thyme, and cook for 15 more minutes.

6. Serve with a sprinkling of Parmesan cheese.

Yield: Makes 8 1-cup servings

Each serving has approximately 146 calories, 11.3 g. protein, 1 g. total fat (0.4 g. unsaturated fat, 0.4 g. saturated fat), 24.4 g. carbohydrates, 1 mg. cholesterol, 3.2 g. fiber, 304 mg. sodium, 99 mg. calcium. Exchanges per serving: ⅓ meat, 1 starch, 2 vegetable.

Six-Vegetable Chowder

Colorful bites of six tender vegetables in a creamy, slightly sweet soup. It freezes well, too.

2 cups Basic Chicken Stock (page 86)

3 cups fresh cooked corn kernels or frozen corn kernels, defrosted

1 medium onion, finely chopped

4 garlic cloves, finely chopped

1 celery stalk without leaves, finely diced

1 potato, peeled and diced

1 cup shredded zucchini

1 medium carrot, peeled and finely diced

1 red bell pepper, seeded and finely chopped

1 can (12-ounce) evaporated skim milk

½ teaspoon freshly ground pepper

1 tablespoon tamari or ⅓ teaspoon salt

1 tablespoon chopped fresh marjoram or 1 teaspoon dried

1⅓ tablespoons chopped fresh dill or 2 teaspoons dried dill

1. In a blender or food processor combine 1 cup of the stock with half the corn and blend until smooth. Pour into a 2-quart soup pot.

2. Cook the onion, garlic, and celery in the corn liquid for 5 minutes over medium heat. Add the diced potato, zucchini, carrot, bell pepper, and the remaining stock and corn. Simmer, covered, for 20 minutes, or until the potatoes and carrots are tender. Add the evaporated skim milk and seasonings. Continue cooking for 5 minutes.

Yield: Makes 8 1-cup servings

Each serving has approximately 124 calories, 7.4 g. protein, 1 g. total fat (0.7 g. unsaturated fat, 0.2 g. saturated fat), 23.8 g. carbohydrates, 1.9 mg. cholesterol, 3.8 g. fiber, 175 mg. sodium, 161 mg. calcium. Exchanges per serving: 1 starch, 1 vegetable, ¼ milk.

Succotash Soup

Here's a golden thyme-flavored soup with lots to bite into — crunchy corn, chewy lima beans, tender sweet potatoes, and chunks of ham-flavored turkey.

1 sweet potato (4 ounces)	1 cup frozen lima beans,
1 medium onion (4 ounces),	defrosted
chopped	½ teaspoon salt
3 cups Basic Chicken Stock	½ teaspoon freshly ground
(page 86)	pepper
2½ cups fresh or frozen corn	1½ tablespoons chopped fresh
kernels	thyme or ½ teaspoon dried
2½ ounces cooked turkey ham,	
cut into small cubes	

1. Preheat oven to 400° F., and bake the sweet potato for 1 hour, or pierce the skin with a fork and microwave it on high, uncovered, for 11 to 13 minutes.

2. Meanwhile, in a 2½-quart saucepan, cook the onion in 3 table-spoons of the chicken stock until the onion is transparent.

3. Add the corn, turkey ham, lima beans, sweet potato meat, and the remaining chicken stock. Simmer for 5 minutes. Season with salt, pepper, and thyme. Cook for 5 additional minutes.

Yield: Makes 8 ¾-cup servings

Each serving has approximately 104 calories, 6.5 g. protein, 1.2 g. total fat (0.7 g. unsaturated fat, 0.3 g. saturated fat), 18.8 g. carbohydrates, 5 mg. cholesterol, 4.7 g. fiber, 250 mg. sodium, 18.6 mg. calcium. Exchanges per serving: ⅓ meat, ⅔ starch, 1 vegetable.

Cream of Broccoli Soup

Crunchy broccoli in a lightly spiced, creamy soup.

4	teaspoons margarine	2⅔	cups skim milk
¾	cup finely chopped onion (1 medium)	1	can (12-ounce) evaporated skim milk
2	large garlic cloves, finely chopped	¾	teaspoon salt
1⅓	pounds trimmed broccoli stems and florets (1 large bunch broccoli)	⅔	teaspoon ground white pepper
		1	teaspoon ground coriander

1. In a heavy 2-quart saucepan melt the margarine, then add the onion and garlic and cook for 2 minutes. Add the broccoli and both milks, and cook over low heat for 25 minutes.

Or combine the margarine, onion, garlic, broccoli, and milks in a microwave-safe dish and cook in a microwave on high for 10 minutes.

2. In a blender or food processor puree the soup in batches, then transfer it to a 2½-quart saucepan. Stir in the salt, pepper, and ground coriander. Heat slowly for 3 minutes, and serve.

Yield: Makes 8 ¾-cup servings

Each serving has approximately 106 calories, 8.4 g. protein, 2.6 g. total fat (1.7 g. unsaturated fat, 0.6 g. saturated fat), 14.3 g. carbohydrates, 3 mg. cholesterol, 2.8 g. fiber, 334 mg. sodium, 266 mg. calcium. Exchanges per serving: ½ fat, ¾ milk, 1 vegetable.

Creamy Orange Carrot Soup

This creamy-tasting soup combines the sweetness of carrots, the gentle tang of oranges, and the crunch of nuts.

1 medium onion, finely chopped	⅔ cup orange juice
2 cups Basic Chicken Stock (page 86)	1 can (12-ounce) evaporated skim milk
2½ cups peeled sliced carrots (about 5 medium carrots)	¾ cup skim milk
1 potato (6 ounces), peeled and cut into 1-inch cubes	½ teaspoon ground white pepper
	2 tablespoons ground hazel-nuts or almonds
	8 sprigs of fresh thyme

1. In a 2-quart saucepan cook the onion in 3 tablespoons of the stock over medium heat until the onion is soft, about 2 to 3 minutes.

2. Add the carrots, potato cubes, orange juice, and remaining stock. Bring to a boil, then simmer, covered, for 25 minutes, or until the carrots and potatoes are tender.

3. In a blender or food processor, puree the soup in two or three batches, adding some of the evaporated milk and skim milk to each batch. The soup should be smooth and creamy. Transfer the pureed soup to a large bowl. When all the soup is pureed, return it to the saucepan and season it with pepper to taste.

4. Reheat the soup before serving, and garnish each individual soup bowl with a sprinkling of ground nuts and a sprig of thyme.

Yield: Makes 8 ¾-cup servings

Each serving has approximately 110 calories, 6.3 g. protein, 1.5 g. total fat (1.1 g. unsaturated fat, 0.2 g. saturated fat), 18.4 g. carbohydrates, 2 mg. cholesterol, 2.5 g. fiber, 107 mg. sodium, 192 mg. calcium.
Exchanges per serving: ⅛ fat, ⅕ fruit, ½ milk, ⅕ starch, 1 vegetable.

Cream of Spinach Soup

Thick, creamy soup flecked with morsels of spinach.

1	leek, split lengthwise, washed, and chopped	2	cups Basic Chicken Stock (page 86)
2	large garlic cloves, chopped	2½	cups evaporated skim milk
2	tablespoons sherry	½	teaspoon salt
1	potato (6 ounces), peeled and cubed	¼	teaspoon white pepper
1	bag (10-ounce) fresh spinach, rinsed well	dash	nutmeg

1. Cook the leek and garlic in the sherry at medium heat for 3 minutes. Add the potato cubes, half the spinach, and the stock. Cover and bring to a boil, then simmer for 15 minutes, or until the potato is tender.

2. In a blender or food processor, puree half the cooked mixture with half the evaporated milk until smooth, then transfer the puree to a large bowl. Repeat with the remaining cooked mixture and milk. Return the entire puree to the pot after blending.

3. Chop the remaining spinach into small pieces and add to the pot. Bring to a boil, and add salt, pepper, and nutmeg. Serve.

Yield: Makes 8 ¾-cup servings

Each serving has approximately 105 calories, 8.4 g. protein, 0.4 g. total fat (0.2 g. unsaturated fat, 0.1 g. saturated fat), 16.4 g. carbohydrates, 3.1 mg. cholesterol, 1.8 g. fiber, 269 mg. sodium, 276 mg. calcium. Exchanges per serving: 2 vegetable, ⅔ milk.

Herbed Tomato Soup

Creamy tomato flavor with the slightly salty bite of Parmesan cheese.

1 small onion, finely chopped	2 tablespoons chopped fresh parsley
2 garlic cloves, finely chopped	1 tablespoon chopped fresh dill
1 can (28-ounce) crushed tomatoes with basil	¾ teaspoon freshly ground black pepper
1 cup tomato juice	2½ tablespoons grated Parmesan cheese
1 can (12-ounce) evaporated skim milk	
2 tablespoons chopped fresh basil	

1. In a 3-quart saucepan cook the onion and garlic in ½ cup of the crushed tomatoes over low heat for 2 minutes. Stir in the rest of the crushed tomatoes, the tomato juice, evaporated milk, basil, parsley, dill, and pepper, and simmer on very low heat for 10 minutes.

2. Puree the soup in a blender or food processor, 2 cups at a time. Sprinkle each serving of soup with some Parmesan cheese.

Yield: Makes 8 ¾-cup servings

Each serving has approximately 87 calories, 7 g. protein, 0.9 g. total fat (0.3 g. unsaturated fat, 0.4 g. saturated fat), 13.7 g. carbohydrates, 3.8 mg. cholesterol, 1.7 g. fiber, 226 mg. sodium, 248 mg. calcium. Exchanges per serving: ⅔ milk, 1 vegetable.

Sweet Potato Soup

Here's a sweet and creamy rich-tasting soup with virtually no fat and only 83 calories a serving. And it's delicious hot or cold.

1½ pounds sweet potatoes or yams, peeled and diced	¼ teaspoon freshly ground pepper
1 medium onion, chopped	½ teaspoon salt
1 celery stalk, chopped	1 cup evaporated skim milk
1½ quarts Basic Chicken Stock (page 86)	

1. In a covered 4-quart soup pot, simmer the sweet potatoes, onion, and celery in the stock for 30 minutes.

2. Stir in the pepper, salt, and evaporated milk. Remove from heat and let soup cool slightly.

3. In a blender or food processor puree the soup in batches until smooth. Reheat the soup if serving warm.

Yield: Makes 8 1-cup servings

Each serving has approximately 83 calories, 5.8 g. protein, 0.2 g. total fat (0.1 g. unsaturated fat, 0.1 g. saturated fat), 14 g. carbohydrates, 1.3 mg. cholesterol, 1.4 g. fiber, 217 mg. sodium, 106 mg. calcium. Exchanges per serving: ½ starch, ½ vegetable, ¼ milk, ⅓ meat.

Pumpkin Soup

A smooth, creamy soup with the deep rich taste of ham-flavored turkey.

1 tablespoon margarine	4 cups Basic Chicken Stock
1 small onion, finely chopped	(page 86)
3 large garlic cloves, chopped	1½ cups canned pumpkin puree
2 ounces turkey ham, finely	⅔ teaspoon salt
chopped	⅔ teaspoon ground black pepper

1. In a 2½-quart saucepan, melt the margarine, then sauté the onion, garlic, and turkey ham until the onion turns translucent.

2. Add the chicken stock and the pumpkin puree. Cook for 5 minutes, uncovered.

3. Add the salt and pepper, and simmer for 5 minutes.

Yield: Makes 8 ¾-cup servings

Each serving has approximately 51 calories, 3.9 g. protein, 2 g. total fat (1.3 g. unsaturated fat, 0.5 g. saturated fat), 5.1 g. carbohydrates, 4 mg. cholesterol, 1.1 g. fiber, 288 mg. sodium, 19.6 mg. calcium. Exchanges per serving: ¼ fat, ⅓ meat, 1 vegetable.

Beef Stock

Rich beef stock to use in sauces and stews.

2½	pounds beef bones	5	celery tops
4	quarts water	2	whole onions
5	whole anise seeds	12	peppercorns

1. In an 8-quart stock pot combine all the ingredients and simmer for 1½ hours, uncovered.
2. Strain through a colander.

Yield: Makes about 2½ quarts

Each serving has approximately 16 calories, 3.6 g. protein, 0 g. total fat (0 g. unsaturated fat, 0 g. saturated fat), 0 g. carbohydrates, 0 mg. cholesterol, 0 g. fiber, 65 mg. sodium, 0.3 mg. calcium.

Exchanges per serving: ⅓ meat.

French Onion Soup

5	cups sliced onions (5 medium onions)	3½	tablespoons low-sodium soy sauce
3	tablespoons sherry	¾	teaspoon freshly ground black pepper
1	tablespoon margarine	½	cup grated Parmesan cheese (2 ounces)
1	tablespoon unbleached flour		
6	cups Beef Stock (above)		

1. In a large heavy-gauge soup pot sauté the onions, dry, for about 2 minutes. When the bottom of the pot begins to brown, add the sherry and continue to sauté the onions for 4 more minutes.
2. Move the onions to a side, and melt the margarine in pot. Sprinkle the flour over the margarine and stir the margarine-flour mixture. Slowly add 1 cup of the beef broth into the margarine-flour mixture, stirring as mixture thickens slightly. Combine the liquid with the cooked onions.
3. Add the remaining 5 cups of the stock, soy sauce, and pepper, and simmer for 15 minutes. Serve with 1 tablespoon of grated Parmesan cheese.

Yield: Makes 8 ¾-cup servings

Each serving has approximately 74 calories, 4.5 g. protein, 1.8 g. total fat (1.2 g. unsaturated fat, 0.3 g. saturated fat), 9 g. carbohydrates, 0 mg. cholesterol, 1.7 g. fiber, 320 mg. sodium, 34 mg. calcium. Exchanges per serving: ¾ meat, 1½ vegetable.

Sweet and Sour Beef and Cabbage Soup

Chewy cabbage strips and beef cubes in a tart but sweet soup that is filling enough to be a main course.

3 garlic cloves, finely chopped	2 cups crushed canned tomatoes
1 medium onion, finely chopped	6 tablespoons lemon juice
4 carrots, peeled, cut into 1-inch chunks	(1½ lemons)
3 celery stalks, cut into 1-inch slices	3 tablespoons brown sugar
	2 tablespoons chopped fresh dill
5 cups Beef Stock (page 98)	½ teaspoon fresh thyme
½ head cabbage, shredded (about 1 pound)	½ teaspoon salt
	1 teaspoon freshly ground pepper
½ pound lean sirloin, trimmed of fat and cut into 1-inch cubes	

1. In a 4-quart soup pot cook the garlic, onion, carrots, celery, and ½ cup of the beef stock for 5 minutes.

2. Add the cabbage, beef cubes, and the remaining 5½ cups of beef stock, and simmer for 15 minutes.

3. Add the tomatoes, lemon juice, brown sugar, dill, thyme, salt, and pepper, and cook for 20 minutes.

Yield: Makes 8 1-cup servings

Each serving has approximately 108 calories, 8 g. protein, 1.6 g. total fat (0.7 g. unsaturated fat, 0.6 g. saturated fat), 17 g. carbohydrates, 10.4 mg. cholesterol, 3.8 g. fiber, 226 mg. sodium, 65 mg. calcium. Exchanges per serving: ⅔ meat, ¼ starch, 2 vegetable.

Basic Fish Stock

A flavorful base for fish chowders and poaching fish.

10 cups water	12 peppercorns
1¼ pounds fish heads, tails, and bones	12 fennel seeds
	12 coriander seeds
2 medium onions	½ cup parsley sprigs, packed
1 carrot	2 garlic cloves
2 celery stalks	

1. Combine all the ingredients in a 4-quart pot. Bring to a low boil, then simmer for 1 hour, uncovered, skimming the surface periodically to remove "film."

2. Strain the stock through a colander into a plastic container, cover, and refrigerate or freeze.

Yield: Makes 7 cups

One cup has approximately 16 calories, 3.6 g. protein, 0 g. total fat (0 g. unsaturated fat, 0 g. saturated fat), 0 g. carbohydrates, 0 mg. cholesterol, 0 g. fiber, 65 mg. sodium, 0 mg. calcium.
Exchanges per cup: ⅓ meat.

Fish Chowder

Add a salad and a slice of grainy bread to this creamy, chunky soup, and you have a splendid meal.

¾ pound baking potatoes	¾ pound scrod or cod fillets, all bones removed
1 medium onion, chopped	
2 garlic cloves, minced	¾ pound catfish fillets
¼ cup white wine	1 cup evaporated skim milk
2 large carrots, peeled and cut into 1-inch pieces	1½ tablespoons chopped fresh dill
2 celery stalks, cut into ½-inch slices	1 tablespoon chopped parsley
	½ tablespoon chopped fresh thyme or ½ teaspoon dried
1 yellow bell pepper, seeded and cut into ¼-inch cubes	¾ teaspoon salt
3 cups Basic Fish Stock (above)	½ teaspoon freshly ground pepper

1. Peel the potatoes, cut into cubes, and cook in 3 cups of water until fork-tender, about 15 – 18 minutes. Drain.

2. In a large soup pot, sauté the onion, garlic, and wine until the onion softens, about 2 minutes.

3. Add the carrots, celery, bell pepper, ⅔ of the cooked potato cubes, and the fish stock. Simmer for 5 minutes, uncovered, over very low heat.

4. Add the fish and evaporated milk, and cook for 5 minutes, uncovered, over medium-low heat.

5. Ladle 2 cups of the broth, ¼ cup of fish pieces, and the remaining ⅓ of the cooked potato cubes into a blender, leaving the carrots, celery, bell pepper, and the rest of the potatoes in the pot. Puree to a creamy consistency, then return to the soup pot. This will thicken the soup.

6. Add the dill, parsley, thyme, salt, and pepper, and cook for 2 – 3 more minutes.

Yield: Makes 8 1-cup servings

Each serving has approximately 167 calories, 20.3 g. protein, 2.4 g. total fat (1.4 g. unsaturated fat, 0.6 g. saturated fat), 14.3 g. carbohydrates, 44.2 mg. cholesterol, 1.7 g. fiber, 329 mg. sodium, 145 mg. calcium.

Exchanges per serving: ¼ starch, 2 meat, 1 vegetable.

Tomato Clam Soup

A smooth, spicy soup with bits of clams for taste and texture.

½ medium onion, chopped
1 garlic clove, finely chopped
½ tablespoon olive oil
1 can (6½-ounce) minced clams
1 can (24-ounce) tomato vegetable juice

1 can (8-ounce) unsalted tomato sauce
10 ounces unsalted clam juice
2 teaspoons fresh rosemary or 1 teaspoon dry
½ teaspoon freshly ground black pepper

1. In a large pot sauté the onion and garlic in the oil over medium-low heat for 3 minutes. Add the remaining ingredients, and simmer for 10 minutes.

Yield: Makes 8 ¾-cup servings

Each serving has approximately 50 calories, 4.7 g. protein, 1.2 g. total fat (0.9 g. unsaturated fat, 0.2 g. saturated fat), 6 g. carbohydrates, 8 mg. cholesterol, 1 g. fiber, 358 mg. sodium, 27 mg. calcium. Exchanges per serving: ½ meat, 1 vegetable.

Chilled Blueberry Soup

Cold soups are one of the delights of warm weather dining, especially if they are sweet, fruity, and creamy.

2¾ cups fresh or frozen unsweetened blueberries, defrosted
3¼ cups plain, non-fat yogurt

2 teaspoons vanilla extract
2 envelopes non-nutritive sweetener

1. In a blender or a food processor, puree all ingredients in batches until smooth. Refrigerate until serving.

Yield: Makes 8 ¾-cup servings

Each serving has approximately 81 calories, 5.6 g. protein, 0.36 g. total fat (0.13 g. unsaturated fat, 0.12 g. saturated fat), 14.4 g. carbohydrates, 1.6 mg. cholesterol, 1.3 g. fiber, 73 mg. sodium, 187 mg. calcium.

Exchanges per serving: ⅔ fruit, ½ milk.

Cold Creamy Cucumber Soup

Very creamy, very filling, very refreshing, especially on a hot day — and a 74-calorie bargain.

2 medium cucumbers, peeled, seeded and cubed (about 4 cups)	½ teaspoon freshly ground pepper
1 cup non-fat buttermilk	4 teaspoons fresh chopped coriander
1 cup non-fat yogurt	
2 scallions, cut into 1-inch pieces	

1. In batches, puree the cucumber with the buttermilk, yogurt, and scallions. Add the pepper. Refrigerate until serving. Garnish each serving with a teaspoon of chopped coriander.

Yield: Makes 4 1-cup servings

Each serving has approximately 74 calories, 6.2 g. protein, 0.4 g. total fat (0.2 g. unsaturated fat, 0.2 g. saturated fat), 12 g. carbohydrates, 2 mg. cholesterol, 2 g. fiber, 78 mg. sodium, 213 mg. calcium.

Exchanges per serving: 1 vegetable, ½ milk.

Salads

Spinach Salad with Smoked
  Oysters and Orange
  Vinaigrette Dressing
Salmon Salad
Hearts of Palm Salad with
  Shrimp
Spicy Lemon Chicken Salad
Fruited Curried Chicken Salad
Poached Chicken Salad with
  Raspberry Vinaigrette
Black Bean Confetti Salad
White Bean Salad with
  Tomato Basil Vinaigrette
Thai Salad with Spicy Dressing

Italian Antipasto Salad
Boston Bibb Salad with
  Roquefort and Apples
Caesar Salad
Spicy Bean Sprout Salad
Creamy Cucumber and Onions
Endive Radicchio Flower
  Salad with Starfruit
Marinated Radishes
Creamy Cole Slaw
Black Cherry Cranberry Mold
Pear and Potato Salad
Mexican Pasta Salad
Orzo Salad

Spinach Salad with Smoked Oysters and Orange Vinaigrette Dressing

Exotic flavors and crunchy textures combined in an unusual salad.

10 ounces fresh spinach, washed and drained well

3½ tablespoons walnuts, coarsely chopped

1 medium red bell pepper, seeded, quartered, and cut into thin strips

1 can (11-ounce) mandarin oranges, gently rinsed of excess sugar and drained

¾ medium red onion, sliced thin

1 can (3.8-ounce) smoked oysters, drained (save oil for dressing)

2 egg whites, hard-boiled and finely chopped (discard yolk)

Dressing:

⅓ cup frozen orange juice concentrate, defrosted

⅓ cup rice vinegar

1 cup water
oil from smoked oysters

1. In a salad bowl combine and toss all the salad ingredients.
2. In a small bowl or pitcher, combine all the dressing ingredients. Serve on the side.

Yield: Serves 8

Each serving has approximately 93 calories, 4 g. protein, 2.6 g. total fat (2 g. unsaturated fat, 0.3 g. saturated fat), 15.4 g. carbohydrates, 7.4 mg. cholesterol, 2.5 g. fiber, 59 mg. sodium, 56 mg. calcium. Exchanges per serving: ½ fat, ¼ fruit, ½ meat, 1 vegetable.

Salmon Salad

Both the pungent flavor and the bite come from capers.

2 cans (7-ounce) red salmon	1 cup chopped celery
2 tablespoons reduced-calorie mayonnaise	2 tablespoons capers
2 tablespoons plain non-fat yogurt	1/8 teaspoon freshly ground pepper
	lettuce

1. Discard the salmon liquid and carefully remove all bones and skin. Crumble the fish coarsely in a 1-quart bowl.
2. Combine the remaining ingredients, and toss with the salmon. Serve on a bed of lettuce.

Yield: Makes 4 ⅔-cup servings

Each serving has approximately 172 calories, 20.2 g. protein, 8.5 g. total fat (5.9 g. unsaturated fat, 2 g. saturated fat), 2.2 g. carbohydrates, 52.8 mg. cholesterol, 0.5 g. fiber, 740 mg. sodium, 237 mg. calcium.

Exchanges per serving: 3 meat.

Hearts of Palm Salad with Shrimp

A beautifully composed salad of chewy seafood and crunchy vegetables arranged on soft lettuce and dressed with a sweet vinaigrette.

1 head Boston Bibb or green leaf lettuce	16 large shrimp
1 can (14-ounce) hearts of palm, drained	12 cherry tomatoes, cut in half
	1 cup Rosy Vinaigrette (page 121)
16 spears fresh, medium-sized asparagus, ends trimmed (about 1 pound	

1. Wash the lettuce, and dry well.
2. Cut each heart of palm into 4 pieces, lengthwise.
3. Steam the asparagus for 3 minutes, or microwave on high for 1 minute, covered.

4. Poach the shrimp in their shells in 4 cups of simmering water for 5 minutes, then cool, shell, and devein them.

5. Toss the cooked seafood in ½ cup of the dressing. Set aside.

6. On each salad plate arrange 3 lettuce leaves. Over them lay 4 pieces of hearts of palm in a crisscross pattern, and 4 asparagus stalks between each heart of palm. Group 4 shrimp and 3 cherry tomatoes decoratively on each plate. Serve extra dressing on the side.

Yield: Serves 4

Each serving has approximately 155 calories, 16.2 g. protein, 7 g. total fat (5 g. unsaturated fat, 1 g. saturated fat), 21.7 g. carbohydrates, 86 mg. cholesterol, 4 g. fiber, 98 mg. sodium, 85 mg. calcium.
Exchanges per serving: 1 fat, ½ meat, 3½ vegetable.

Spicy Lemon Chicken Salad

Tender chewy chicken bites marinated in a spicy hot and tartly citrus sauce.

½ cup Spicy Lemon Dipping Sauce (page 132)

1½ tablespoons chopped fresh cilantro

2 cups cooked, skinless chicken (10 ounces total, white and dark meat), shredded into small pieces

1 head Bibb lettuce

½ cup shredded carrots

1. Combine lemon dipping sauce and cilantro, and marinate chicken pieces in it for 15 minutes.

2. Line 4 salad plates with lettuce leaves. Place ½ cup of chicken on each plate, and drizzle the excess marinade on top. Garnish with shredded carrots.

Yield: Serves 4

Each serving has approximately 162 calories, 19.5 g. protein, 6.5 g. total fat (3.8 g. unsaturated fat, 1.8 g. saturated fat), 6 g. carbohydrates, 57 mg. cholesterol, 1.3 g. fiber, 204 mg. sodium, 36.5 mg. calcium.
Exchanges per serving: 2 meat, ⅙ starch, 1 vegetable.

Fruited Curried Chicken Salad

Chunky chicken and crisp fruits bathed in a light curry dressing.

2 cups skinless, boneless, cooked chicken cut into chunks (about 10 ounces)	2 tablespoons reduced-calorie mayonnaise
1½ cups apple cut into ¼-inch cubes (about 1 medium apple)	2 tablespoons finely chopped onion
¼ cup canned unsweetened crushed pineapple	1 teaspoon curry powder
	½ teaspoon sugar
¼ cup plain non-fat yogurt	¼ teaspoon salt
	¼ teaspoon pepper

1. In a large bowl combine the chicken, apple cubes, and pineapple, and set aside.

2. In another bowl combine the remaining ingredients and mix well. Pour the salad dressing over the chicken mixture and toss.

Yield: Makes 4 ⅔-cup servings

Each serving has approximately 200 calories, 21.3 g. protein, 8 g. total fat (5.2 g. unsaturated fat, 2 g. saturated fat), 10.3 g. carbohydrates, 65.2 mg. cholesterol, 1.4 g. fiber, 262 mg. sodium, 47.3 mg. calcium. Exchanges per serving: ⅔ fruit, 2½ meat.

Poached Chicken Salad with Raspberry Vinaigrette

Strips of tender chicken, slices of crunchy, sweet sunchokes, and the snappy bite of arugula in a light and fruity vinaigrette.

3 cups Basic Chicken Stock (page 86)	½ pint fresh raspberries
½ teaspoon salt	1 tablespoon olive oil
3 sprigs of fresh marjoram or tarragon	2 tablespoons raspberry vinegar
	1 tablespoon water
12 ounces boneless, skinless chicken breasts, fat removed	½ head Bibb lettuce leaves, washed and dried
½ pound Jerusalem artichokes (sunchokes)	1 bunch fresh arugula leaves, washed and dried

1. In a 10-inch sauté pan bring the chicken broth, salt, and marjoram or tarragon to a low simmer. Turn heat as low as possible, and poach the chicken breasts in the warm broth for 6 minutes. Remove the chicken with a slotted spoon and set aside to cool. Use the broth for soup, or discard it.

2. Wash and dry the sunchokes, then cut them into ⅛-inch slices. Carefully rinse the raspberries and drain off excess water.

3. Cut the chicken into strips about 3 to 4 inches long and ⅓ inch wide.

4. In a blender or food processor combine the olive oil, vinegar, water, and ¼ cup of the raspberries, and puree until smooth.

5. On each salad plate lay some Bibb lettuce and arugula, top with strips of chicken, slices of sunchoke, and the remaining whole raspberries. Spoon the raspberry vinaigrette on top, or serve on the side.

Yield: Serves 4

Each serving has approximately 191 calories, 22 g. protein, 4.7 g. total fat (3.4 g. unsaturated fat, 0.8 g. saturated fat), 15.7 g. carbohydrates, 49 mg. cholesterol, 3.4 g. fiber, 332 mg. sodium, 54 mg. calcium. Exchanges per serving: ¼ fat, ¼ fruit, 2 meat, 2 vegetable.

Black Bean Confetti Salad

Crunchy, colorful, and slightly tart.

1 cup dried black beans	1 large garlic clove, finely chopped
½ cup frozen corn kernels, defrosted	2 scallions, sliced ½-inch thick
⅓ pound plum tomatoes, cut into eighths	¼ cup lime juice (about 2 limes)
1 celery stalk, thinly sliced	¼ teaspoon salt
2 tablespoons chopped cilantro	½ teaspoon coarsely ground pepper

1. Bring 3 cups of water to a boil and remove from heat. Meanwhile pick through the black beans to remove any small stones.

2. Soak the beans in 3 cups of boiled water for one hour. Drain through a colander.

3. In a 2½-quart pot, bring 1½ quarts of water to a boil. Add the

beans, reduce heat, and simmer for 1 hour, or until the beans are tender. Drain through a colander after cooking.

4. In a medium-sized bowl combine the beans with the remaining ingredients, and mix well. Serve chilled.

Yield: Makes 8 ½-cup servings

Each serving has approximately 72.8 calories, 4.4 g. protein, 0.4 g. total fat (0.25 g. unsaturated fat, 0.09 g. saturated fat), 14 g. carbohydrates, 0 mg. cholesterol, 4.7 g. fiber, 74.5 mg. sodium, 18.3 mg. calcium.

Exchanges per serving: ¾ starch, ½ vegetable.

White Bean Salad with Tomato Basil Vinaigrette

Here's a tender salad as colorful as the Italian flag, gently bathed in a zingy herb vinaigrette.

Salad:

- 3 cups fresh broccoli florets
- 1 can (19-ounce) white beans (about 2 cups cooked beans)
- ¼ cup fresh basil leaves, packed
- 1 cup chopped tomatoes (about 2 small tomatoes)

Dressing:

- ½ tablespoon corn oil
- 2 tablespoons red wine vinegar
- ¼ cup fresh basil leaves
- 2 tablespoons tomato juice
- ¼ teaspoon salt
- ¼ teaspoon ground black pepper

1. Steam the broccoli for 2 minutes. Immediately rinse the broccoli under cold water in a colander to stop the cooking. Set the broccoli aside.

   To microwave: Place the broccoli in a microwave-safe dish, add 1 tablespoon water, cover tightly with plastic wrap, and cook on high for 3 minutes. Immediately rinse the broccoli under cold water in a colander to stop the cooking.

2. Place the beans in a colander and drain under cold water to remove excess starch.

3. Tear the basil into small pieces.

4. In a serving dish combine the broccoli, beans, basil, and tomatoes.

5. In a blender or food processor, combine the dressing ingredients and puree until smooth. Pour over the salad and toss well.

Yield: Makes 4 1½-cup servings

Each serving has approximately 182 calories, 11.1 g. protein, 3 g. total fat (2.0 g. unsaturated fat, 0.4 g. saturated fat), 32 g. carbohydrates, 0 mg. cholesterol, 10.8 g. fiber, 160 mg. sodium, 198 mg. calcium. Exchanges per serving: ½ fat, 1⅔ starch, 1 vegetable.

Thai Salad with Spicy Dressing

A beautifully arranged salad with crisp, juicy vegetables, crunchy nuts, and a very spicy dressing.

1 head romaine lettuce, leaves washed, dried, and lightly shredded

4 ripe Italian plum tomatoes, cut into eighths

4 hard-boiled egg whites, sliced (yolk discarded)

1 large cucumber, sliced

2 medium carrots, shredded

2 tablespoons finely chopped peanuts

1 cup fresh mung bean sprouts

1 recipe Spicy Lemon Dipping Sauce (page 132)

1. On 4 salad plates, arrange the romaine leaves. Place the tomato slices in spoke-fashion on the lettuce, and the sliced egg whites and cucumbers on top. Spoon the grated carrot in the center, and sprinkle the grated peanuts and mung bean sprouts over the composed salad.

2. Serve each salad with 2 tablespoons Spicy Lemon Dipping Sauce.

Yield: Serves 4

Each serving has approximately 119 calories, 7.3 g. protein, 3 g. total fat (2.2 g. unsaturated fat, 0.4 g. saturated fat), 19.4 g. carbohydrates, 0 mg. cholesterol, 7.3 g. fiber, 199 mg. sodium, 99 mg. calcium. Exchanges per serving: 1 meat, ⅙ starch, 2 vegetable.

Italian Antipasto Salad

A colorful and unusual antipasto vegetable salad with a variety of tastes and textures.

1 tablespoon extra-virgin olive oil	1 cup fresh fennel root, thinly sliced
2 tablespoons balsamic vinegar	⅓ pound plum tomatoes, cut into eighths
1 large red bell pepper, cut into long, thin strips	8 pitted black olives, cut in half
½ cup lightly chopped basil leaves	2 ounces pepperoncini, rinsed and cut in half lengthwise
3 canned artichoke hearts, drained and cut in quarters	½ head radicchio lettuce

1. In a medium-sized bowl, mix the olive oil and vinegar. Add the red pepper slices, basil, artichoke hearts, fennel slices, plum tomatoes, olive halves, and pepperoncini, and toss together gently.

2. Line individual plates with radicchio leaves. Top with the dressed vegetables.

Yield: Serves 4

Each serving has approximately 69 calories, 2.2 g. protein, 4.5 g. total fat (3.4 g. unsaturated fat, 0.7 g. saturated fat), 8 g. carbohydrates, 0 mg. cholesterol, 4.7 g. fiber, 282 mg. sodium, 67 mg. calcium. Exchanges per serving: ¾ fat, 1½ vegetable.

Boston Bibb Salad with Roquefort and Apples

The soft texture of Bibb lettuce with crisp apple bites and slightly salty Roquefort, in a fruity dressing.

1 head Boston Bibb lettuce	1 tablespoon olive or walnut oil
1 Granny Smith apple, chopped into small pieces	1½ tablespoons raspberry vinegar
1 ounce Roquefort or other blue cheese, crumbled	¼ teaspoon coarse black pepper

1. Wash the lettuce and drain well in a colander or salad spinner. Tear into bite-sized pieces, and transfer to a large serving bowl.

2. Add the chopped apples and crumbled blue cheese, and toss to combine. Add the oil, vinegar, and black pepper, and toss.

Yield: Serves 4

Each serving has approximately 87 calories, 2.7 g. protein, 5.7 g. total fat (3.5 g. unsaturated fat, 1.8 g. saturated fat), 7.8 g. carbohydrates, 5.2 mg. cholesterol, 2 g. fiber, 103 mg. sodium, 69 mg. calcium. Exchanges per serving: ½ fat, ¼ fruit, ¼ meat, 1½ vegetable.

Caesar Salad

A spirited salad with little cholesterol but a strong garlic punch, crisp lettuce, and the crunch of croutons.

1	head romaine lettuce	¼	cup frozen, liquid, cholesterol-free egg replacement, defrosted
2	small or 1 large garlic clove		
1	tablespoon lemon juice	¼	teaspoon black, ground pepper
¼	teaspoon powdered mustard	1	tablespoon Parmesan cheese
4	anchovies	1	tablespoon vinegar
2	teaspoons olive oil, from anchovy can	4	tablespoons croutons

1. Wash the lettuce and dry the leaves well. Tear into 1- to 2-inch pieces, and transfer to a salad bowl.

2. Using a food processor or mortar and pestle, puree or pulverize the garlic. Add the lemon juice, mustard, anchovies, oil, liquid egg replacement, pepper, Parmesan cheese, and vinegar, and mix well.

3. Just before serving, toss the romaine with the dressing, and top with croutons.

Yield: Serves 4

Each serving has approximately 79 calories, 4.8 g. protein, 4.8 g. total fat (3.5 g. unsaturated fat, 0.9 g. saturated fat), 5 g. carbohydrates, 4 mg. cholesterol, 1.5 g. fiber, 90 mg. sodium, 71 mg. calcium. Exchanges per serving: 1 fat, 2 vegetable.

Spicy Bean Sprout Salad

Lots of crunch with a tart bite.

½ pound mung bean sprouts
   (about 4½ cups)
⅔ cup rice vinegar
⅔ cup water
1 tablespoon ground peanuts

1 scallion, sliced
¼ teaspoon chili pepper flakes
2 teaspoons low-sodium soy
   sauce

1. Combine all the ingredients in a bowl, and marinate for 1 hour.
2. Drain through a fine-mesh strainer and discard the marinade.

Yield: Makes 4 ½-cup servings

Each serving has approximately 37 calories, 2.5 g. protein, 1.2 g. total fat (1 g. unsaturated fat, 0.2 g. saturated fat), 6.5 g. carbohydrates, 0 mg. cholesterol, 1.7 g. fiber, 104 mg. sodium, 14.8 mg. calcium. Exchanges per serving: 1 vegetable, ¼ fat.

Creamy Cucumber and Onions

Crisp vegetables bathed in a creamy dill dressing.

¼ cup vinegar
¼ cup water
1 teaspoon sugar
¼ teaspoon ground pepper
1 pound cucumber

¼ pound red onion (about 1
   medium onion)
⅔ cup plain non-fat yogurt
1 tablespoon snipped fresh dill,
   or ¾ teaspoon dried

1. Combine the vinegar, water, sugar, and pepper to make a marinade.
2. Peel the cucumber and cut into ⅛-inch-thick slices. Cut the onion in half, then slice very thin. Add to the marinade, cover, and let marinate for 2 hours.
3. In a large bowl mix the yogurt and dill.
4. Drain the cucumber and onion slices, discarding the marinade, then add to the yogurt dressing and mix well.

Yield: Makes 4 ¾-cup servings

Each serving has approximately 29 calories, 0.8 g. protein, 0.2 g. total fat (0.1 g. unsaturated fat, 0.04 g. saturated fat), 6.5 g. carbohydrates, 0 mg. cholesterol, 1.5 g. fiber, 2.5 mg. sodium, 20 mg. calcium. Exchanges per serving: 1 vegetable.

Endive Radicchio Flower Salad with Starfruit

A beautifully composed salad with a touch of crabmeat, crisp endive, and the slightly bitter taste of radicchio, all drizzled with starfruit dressing.

1 head radicchio lettuce	1 tablespoon walnut or olive oil
1 head Belgian endive lettuce (or 20 leaves)	1 tablespoon water
	2 tablespoons raspberry vinegar
4 sprigs watercress	1 teaspoon fresh marjoram
½ avocado, cut into 20 thin strips	leaves or ½ teaspoon dried
4 ounces fresh, canned, or frozen crabmeat	
3 starfruit	

1. Cut each radicchio leaf into 3 pieces.
2. Cut 1 inch off the roots of the Belgian endive lettuce, and separate the leaves.
3. Arrange 5 radicchio pieces and 5 endive leaves alternately around each of the 4 salad plates, and between each place an avocado slice. Put about 1 teaspoon of crabmeat on each piece of radicchio leaf toward the bottom.
4. Cut two of the starfruit crosswise into 10 slices each, so you can see their star-shape in cross section. Lay five starfruit slices around the rim of each plate, and place a sprig of watercress in the center.
5. In the blender or food processor puree the remaining starfruit with oil, water, vinegar, and marjoram. Drizzle each salad with 1 tablespoon of dressing.

Yield: Serves 4

Each serving has approximately 144 calories, 7.9 g. protein, 8.3 g. total fat (6.3 g. unsaturated fat, 1 g. saturated fat), 12 g. carbohydrates, 28.4 mg. cholesterol, 4.8 g. fiber, 94 mg. sodium, 75 mg. calcium. Exchanges per serving: 1½ fat, 1 meat, 1 vegetable.

Marinated Radishes

Two kinds of radishes in a light, tart, refreshing marinade.

¾ **pound daikon radishes**	½ **cup water**
2 **ounces red radishes**	1½ **teaspoons sugar**
½ **cup rice vinegar**	2 **slices fresh ginger**

1. Peel the daikon radishes, and slice both kinds of radishes very thin.

2. In a bowl combine the vinegar, water, sugar, and ginger for a marinade. Add the radish slices, cover, and refrigerate for 2 hours.

Yield: Makes 4 ¾-cup servings

Each serving has approximately 28 calories, 0.6 g. protein, 0.2 g. total fat (0.1 g. unsaturated fat, 0 g. saturated fat), 7.6 g. carbohydrates, 0 mg. cholesterol, 2.3 g. fiber, 21 mg. sodium, 29 mg. calcium. Exchanges per serving: 1 vegetable.

Creamy Cole Slaw

Here's an old favorite in a creamy low-calorie version, with all its crunch intact.

½ **pound cut, shredded, green cabbage (about 4 cups)**	¼ **cup plain non-fat yogurt**
½ **cup grated carrots (about 1 medium carrot)**	1 **tablespoon apple juice concentrate**
2 **tablespoons reduced-calorie mayonnaise**	¼ **teaspoon coarsely ground pepper**
	1 **tablespoon vinegar**

1. Combine the cabbage and carrots in a large bowl.

2. In another bowl, combine the remaining ingredients. Add to the cabbage mixture and toss well to coat the slaw.

Yield: Makes 8 ½-cup servings

Each serving has approximately 30 calories, 0.8 g. protein, 1.3 g. total fat (1 g. unsaturated fat, 0.3 g. saturated fat), 4.1 g. carbohydrates, 1.4 mg. cholesterol, 0.9 g. fiber, 42 mg. sodium, 29.8 mg. calcium. Exchanges per serving: 1 vegetable, ¼ fat.

Black Cherry Cranberry Mold

A creamy, fruit-flavored gelatin studded with chunks of three fruits.

½ package (28-ounce) cranberries
1 package (12-ounce) frozen
unsweetened dark cherries
1 can (8-ounce) unsweetened
pineapple chunks (retain juice)

1 envelope unflavored gelatin
¼ cup reduced-fat sour cream

1. In a 3-quart saucepan combine the cranberries, cherries, and pineapple chunks, and cook over low heat until the cranberries pop.

2. Put the drained pineapple juice in a small saucepan. Sprinkle the gelatin on top, and let sit for 2 minutes. Then heat over low heat until the gelatin dissolves in the juice. Pour the gelatin into the cranberry-cherry mixture, and stir well.

3. Fold the reduced-calorie sour cream into the fruit mixture, and stir until combined.

4. Pour the fruit mixture into a 1-quart mold or an 8×1¼-inch ring mold. Refrigerate for 2 hours, or until the mixture gels.

Yield: Makes 8 ½-cup servings
Each serving has approximately 99 calories, 2 g. protein, 1.4 g. total fat (0.4 g. unsaturated fat, 0.9 g. saturated fat), 20.7 g. carbohydrates, 0 mg. cholesterol, 2.8 g. fiber, 9 mg. sodium, 13 mg. calcium.
Exchanges per serving: ⅛ fat, 1⅓ fruit.

Pear and Potato Salad

An unusual combination of juicy pear chunks and tender new potatoes in a creamy dressing.

1 pound new potatoes
2 small or 1 large ripe pear, like
Anjou, Bosc, or Comice
1 tablespoon lemon juice
2 celery stalks, finely chopped
2 tablespoons finely chopped
parsley
3 tablespoons finely chopped
raw onion

3 tablespoons plain non-fat
yogurt
2 tablespoons reduced-calorie
mayonnaise
¼ teaspoon freshly ground
pepper

1. Bring 2 quarts of water to a boil. Add the potatoes, and boil for 20 minutes, or until fork-tender.

2. Remove the potatoes from water and let cool.

3. Peel and core the pears, then cut them into ½-inch slices. To prevent the pears from browning, soak them in a cup of water mixed with 1 tablespoon of lemon juice.

4. Combine the celery, parsley, and onion with the yogurt, mayonnaise, and pepper.

5. Slice the potatoes as thin as you can without their falling apart.

6. Remove the pears from the water-lemon solution, and combine with the potatoes and yogurt-mayonnaise mixture. Mix the salad carefully so the potatoes don't crumble.

Yield: Makes 8 ½-cup servings

Each serving has approximately 81 calories, 1.6 g. protein, 1.4 g. total fat (1.1 g. unsaturated fat, 0.3 g. saturated fat), 16 g. carbohydrates, 1.4 mg. cholesterol, 1.7 g. fiber, 45 mg. sodium, 22 mg. calcium. Exchanges per serving: ¼ fat, ¼ fruit, ¾ starch.

Mexican Pasta Salad

Lots of crunch and color in this spicy salad.

2½ quarts water	½ cup cooked fresh corn, or frozen corn kernels, defrosted
6 ounces rigatoni	
1 tablespoon corn oil	10 large black olives, pitted and quartered
¼ red onion, chopped	
3 tablespoons chopped fresh cilantro (coriander)	¼ green bell pepper, chopped
	½ teaspoon crushed red pepper
½ pound cherry tomatoes (about 10 tomatoes), cut in half	¼ teaspoon salt
	2 tablespoons lime juice

1. Bring the water to a boil, and cook the pasta according to package instructions, but without any oil or salt. Drain the cooked pasta in a colander, and rinse with cool water.

2. In a large bowl combine remaining ingredients. Add the cooled pasta, and toss until well combined.

Yield: Makes 8 ⅔-cup servings

Each serving has approximately 126 calories, 3.8 g. protein, 4 g. total fat (2 g. unsaturated fat, 0.7 g. saturated fat), 20 g. carbohydrates, 0 mg. cholesterol, 2.8 g. fiber, 123 mg. sodium, 21.5 mg. calcium. Exchanges per serving: ½ fat, 1 starch, ½ vegetable.

Orzo Salad

Crunchy vegetable bits and rice-shaped pasta in a refreshing salad with oriental flavor.

2 quarts boiling water	2 tablespoons fresh chopped
5 ounces orzo pasta	chives
1 yellow bell pepper, cut into	1 tablespoon toasted sesame oil
⅓-inch squares	1½ tablespoons low-sodium soy
2 ounces snow peas, ends	sauce
trimmed, and cut into	1 tablespoon Szechuan season-
julienne strips	ing sauce
2 medium carrots, peeled and	
diced into ¼-inch pieces	

1. Boil 2 quarts of water. Add the orzo, and cook for 10–12 minutes. Drain through a colander, rinse with cool water, and set aside.

2. In a large bowl combine the bell pepper, snow peas, carrots, and chives. Add the orzo, and mix again.

3. Add the sesame oil, soy sauce, and Szechuan seasoning sauce, and mix well.

Yield: Makes 8 ½-cup servings

Each serving has approximately 100 calories, 3.3 g. protein, 2.5 g. total fat (1.8 g. unsaturated fat, 0.4 g. saturated fat), 16.2 g. carbohydrates, 0 mg. cholesterol, 2.2 g. fiber, 126 mg. sodium, 19 mg. calcium. Exchanges per serving: ½ fat, ¾ starch, ½ vegetable.

Dressings, Dips, Relishes, and Sauces

Cucumber Blue Cheese
    Dressing
Rosy Vinaigrette
Fresh Herb Vinaigrette
Honey Mustard Vinaigrette
Sweet Orange Poppy Dressing
Horseradish Spread
Creamy Yogurt Cheese
Smoked Salmon Spread
Honey Mustard Dip
Creamy Herb Dip
Spinach Dip
Onion Dip
Crabmeat Avocado Dip
Carrot Tofu Dip
Barbecue Sauce
Spicy Salsa
Enchilada Sauce
Green Tomatillo Sauce

Wasabi
Spicy Lemon Dipping Sauce
Pesto Genovese
Peppery Mushroom Sauce
Tartar Sauce
Tomato Anchovy Sauce
Sweet and Sour Tomato Sauce
Creamy Tomato Sauce
Italian Spaghetti Sauce with
    Fresh Herbs
Lemon Sauce
Apple Rhubarb Sauce
Cranberry Ginger Sauce
Mango Cream Sauce
Raspberry Sauce
Bittersweet Chocolate Cherry
    Sauce
Mocha Sauce

Cucumber Blue Cheese Dressing

A creamy, light, low-calorie blue cheese dressing for salads.

½ medium cucumber, peeled, seeded, and cubed (about 1 cup)	¼ cup skim milk ¼ cup plain, non-fat yogurt 1½ ounces blue cheese

1. Puree all the ingredients in a blender or food processor until smooth and creamy.

Yield: Makes 1 cup
One tablespoon has approximately 14 calories, .95 g. protein, .8 g. total fat (0.25 g. unsaturated fat, 0.05 g. saturated fat), .8 g. carbohydrates, 2.1 mg. cholesterol, 0.1 g. fiber, 42 mg. sodium, 26.5 mg. calcium.
Exchanges per serving: ⅙ fat, ¹⁄₁₆ milk.

Rosy Vinaigrette

A lovely dressing for salad greens with the sweet flavor of pimientos.

1 can (7½-ounce) pimientos	6 tablespoons balsamic vinegar
2 tablespoons olive oil	12 tablespoons water

1. Combine all the ingredients in a blender, and puree until smooth.

Yield: Makes 2 cups
One tablespoon has approximately 9 calories, 0.05 g. protein, 0.9 g. total fat (0.7 g. unsaturated fat, 0.1 g. saturated fat), 0.5 g. carbohydrates, 0 mg. cholesterol, 0.1 g. fiber, 0 mg. sodium, 0.5 mg. calcium.
Exchanges per serving: ⅕ fat.

Fresh Herb Vinaigrette

A mélange of three fresh herbs for poached chicken and fish, as well as salad greens.

4 tablespoons white wine vinegar	½ tablespoon fresh basil leaves
1 tablespoon olive oil	½ small clove garlic
3 tablespoons water	⅛ teaspoon salt
½ teaspoon fresh rosemary	⅛ teaspoon freshly ground black pepper
½ teaspoon fresh thyme leaves	

1. Combine all the ingredients in a blender or food processor and puree.

Yield: Makes ½ cup

One tablespoon has approximately 17 calories, 0 g. protein, 1.7 g. total fat (1.4 g. unsaturated fat, 0.2 g. saturated fat), 0.7 g. carbohydrates, 0 mg. cholesterol, 0.1 g. fiber, 34 mg. sodium, 5 mg. calcium. Exchanges per serving: ⅓ fat.

Honey Mustard Vinaigrette

A lovely dressing for greens.

1 tablespoon olive oil	1 clove garlic, peeled
2 tablespoons water	2½ tablespoons balsamic vinegar
2 teaspoons prepared Dijon mustard	2 teaspoons honey

1. Combine all the ingredients in a blender or food processor, and puree for 1 minute.

Yield: Makes ½ cup

One tablespoon has approximately 22 calories, 0.1 g. protein, 1.8 g. total fat (1.4 g. unsaturated fat, 0.2 g. saturated fat), 2 g. carbohydrates, 0 mg. cholesterol, 0 g. fiber, 17 mg. sodium, 2 mg. calcium. Exchanges per serving: ⅓ fat, 1/16 starch.

Sweet Orange Poppy Dressing

A slightly sweet, slightly sour dressing for salads.

⅓ cup frozen orange juice
    concentrate, defrosted
⅓ cup red wine vinegar

⅓ cup water
1 teaspoon poppy seeds

1. Combine all the ingredients in a stoppered 1-cup jar. Store in refrigerator, and shake before using.

Yield: Makes 1 cup
Each 2-tablespoon serving has approximately 22 calories, 0.4 g. protein, 0.2 g. total fat (0.1 g. unsaturated fat, 0 g. saturated fat), 5.1 g. carbohydrates, 0 mg. cholesterol, 0.2 g. fiber, 0.5 mg. sodium, 9.6 mg. calcium.
Exchanges per serving: ⅓ fruit.

Horseradish Spread

A tangy, creamy spread to serve with Smoked Turkey Bites (page 76) or as a dip for raw vegetables.

½ cup Creamy Yogurt Cheese
    (page 124)
1½ tablespoons prepared white
    horseradish

1. Combine the ingredients well in a small bowl or food processor.

Yield: Makes ½ cup
One tablespoon has approximately 15 calories, 1.4 g. protein, 0 g. total fat (0 g. unsaturated fat, 0 g. saturated fat), 2.3 g. carbohydrates, 0.5 mg. cholesterol, 0 g. fiber, 22.6 mg. sodium, 58.2 mg. calcium.
Exchanges per serving: ⅕ milk.

Creamy Yogurt Cheese

A slightly tart and creamy low-calorie version of cream cheese for morning toast, or as a base for many flavored spreads like Horseradish (page 123) and Smoked Salmon (below).

1 quart plain, non-fat yogurt
1 packet non-nutritive sweetener
   (optional)

1. Line a colander with three layers of cheesecloth. Pour the yogurt in and let it drip overnight. Discard the drippings. The mixture will be as thick as cream cheese, and slightly more tart. You may want to add sweetener to taste.

2. Refrigerate in a covered container. The spread will last as long as the date on the yogurt package.

Yield: Makes 2 cups
One tablespoon has approximately 14 calories, 1.4 g. protein, 0 g. total fat (0 g. unsaturated fat, 0 g. saturated fat), 2 g. carbohydrates, 0.5 mg. cholesterol, 0 g. fiber, 20 mg. sodium, 56.5 mg. calcium.
Exchanges per serving: 1/5 milk.

Smoked Salmon Spread

Serve on your morning bagel or on Bagel Chips (page 261).

4   ounces Creamy Yogurt
    Cheese (above)
1½ ounces smoked salmon or
    lox, finely chopped

1. Combine the ingredients in a bowl or food processor.

Yield: Makes ½ cup
One tablespoon has approximately 20 calories, 2.3 g. protein, 0.3 g. total fat (0.2 g. unsaturated fat, 0.1 g. saturated fat), 2 g. carbohydrates, 1.8 mg. cholesterol, 0 g. fiber, 62 mg. sodium, 57 mg. calcium.
Exchanges per serving: ¼ milk.

Honey Mustard Dip

Here's a rich sweet mustard dip, especially good with vegetables.

4 tablespoons stone-ground
  mustard
1 tablespoon honey
4 tablespoons plain non-fat
  yogurt

2 teaspoons chopped fresh
  tarragon or 1 teaspoon dried

1. Combine all the ingredients in a bowl and mix well.

Yield: Makes ½ cup

One tablespoon has approximately 19 calories, 0.9 g. protein, 0.4 g. total fat (0.3 g. unsaturated fat, 0 g. saturated fat), 3.3 g. carbohydrates, 0 mg. cholesterol, 0.06 g. fiber, 105 mg. sodium, 23 mg. calcium.

Exchanges per serving: ⅛ milk, ⅛ starch.

Creamy Herb Dip

A creamy dip for vegetables, redolent with four fresh herbs.

1 cup 1-percent-fat cottage
  cheese
1 teaspoon crumbled fresh
  rosemary
½ teaspoon chopped fresh thyme
1 tablespoon chopped fresh
  chives

1 teaspoon chopped fresh chervil
½ teaspoon freshly ground black
  pepper

1. In the food processor puree the cottage cheese until completely smooth. Add the herbs and pepper, and puree for 15 more seconds.

Yield: Makes 1 cup

Each tablespoon has approximately 11 calories, 1.8 g. protein, 0.2 g. total fat (0.1 g. unsaturated fat, 0.1 g. saturated fat), 0.5 g. carbohydrates, 0.6 mg. cholesterol, 0 g. fiber, 57 mg. sodium, 10 mg. calcium.

Exchanges per serving: ⅛ milk.

Spinach Dip

A low-calorie version of a familiar dip for vegetables or to spread on pumpernickel squares.

10 ounces fresh spinach or frozen spinach, defrosted	2½ tablespoons reduced-calorie mayonnaise
1 small onion, finely chopped	¼ teaspoon freshly ground black pepper
2 garlic cloves, finely chopped	
1 can (6-ounce) minced clams, including juices	1 tablespoon Worcestershire sauce
2 tablespoons plain, non-fat yogurt	¼ teaspoon ground nutmeg

1. Cook the fresh spinach in a sauté pan for 5 minutes, or in a microwave on high for 3 minutes, covered. Drain the fresh or defrosted spinach, squeeze dry in your hands, and chop finely. Set aside.

2. In an 8-inch sauté pan cook the onion and garlic in 1 tablespoon of the clam juice for 2 to 3 minutes. Set aside, and discard the remaining clam juice.

3. In a bowl or a food processor combine all the ingredients, including the spinach and sautéed onion-garlic mixture.

Yield: Makes 2 cups

One tablespoon has approximately 13 calories, 1 g. protein, 0.5 g. total fat (0.4 g. unsaturated fat, 0.1 g. saturated fat), 1 g. carbohydrates, 2.3 mg. cholesterol, 0.4 g. fiber, 30 mg. sodium, 15.3 mg. calcium. Exchanges per serving: ⅛ fat, ¼ vegetable.

Onion Dip

A low-calorie rendition of a favorite dip for fresh vegetables.

¼ cup onion flakes	2 packets low-sodium instant beef bouillon
¼ cup reduced-calorie sour cream	
1½ cups plain non-fat yogurt	¼ packet non-nutritive sweetener (optional)
½ teaspoon salt	

1. Preheat oven to 375° F.
2. Pour the onion flakes into a baking pan, and toast until lightly browned, about 4 or 5 minutes.
3. In a bowl combine the sour cream and yogurt, mixing well with a whisk. Stir in the toasted onion flakes, salt, beef bouillon powder, and sweetener.

Yield: Makes 2 cups
One tablespoon has approximately 11 calories, 0.7 g. protein, 0.4 g. total fat (0.1 g. unsaturated fat, 0.1 g. saturated fat), 1.4 g. carbohydrates, 0.2 mg. cholesterol, 0 g. fiber, 43 mg. sodium, 22.5 mg. calcium.
Exchanges per serving: ⅛ milk.

Crabmeat Avocado Dip

Chewy shreds of crabmeat in a light creamy sauce with a hint of lemon. Serve it as a dip with fresh vegetables, or as a spread.

¼ ripe medium avocado
4 ounces fresh, canned, or frozen and defrosted crabmeat
1 tablespoon plain non-fat yogurt
1 tablespoon reduced-calorie mayonnaise

½ teaspoon freshly ground black pepper
2 tablespoons chopped fresh sorrel or lemon balm

1. In a bowl, lightly chop the avocado with a knife.
2. Stir in the crabmeat, yogurt, mayonnaise, pepper, and chopped herb.

Yield: Makes 1 cup
Each tablespoon has approximately 16 calories, 1.6 g. protein, 0.9 g. total fat (0.7 g. unsaturated fat, 0.2 g. saturated fat), 0.4 g. carbohydrates, 7.4 mg. cholesterol, 0.3 g. fiber, 28 mg. sodium, 10 mg. calcium.
Exchanges per serving: ⅕ fat, ¼ meat.

Carrot Tofu Dip

Creamy and smooth, with a light peanut flavor.

2 medium carrots, peeled and cut into ½-inch slices	1 tablespoon smooth peanut butter
8 ounces soft tofu (silken), drained	1 garlic clove, finely chopped

1. Steam the carrots for 10 minutes or microwave for 5 minutes on high, covered.
2. In a blender or food processor, puree the carrots with the remaining ingredients until smooth, scraping the container sides occasionally.

Yield: Makes 1¼ cups

Each tablespoon has approximately 17 calories, 1.2 g. protein, 1 g. total fat (0.7 g. unsaturated fat, 0.2 g. saturated fat), 1.1 g. carbohydrates, 0 mg. cholesterol, 0.4 g. fiber, 6.6 mg. sodium, 14 mg. calcium. Exchanges per serving: ⅕ fat, ⅒ meat, ⅕ vegetable.

Barbecue Sauce

Sweet, spicy, and hot. Use it with Barbecued Chicken Legs (page 174), and any other barbecue favorite.

1 pound Italian plum tomatoes, cored and seeded	2 tablespoons tomato paste
2 garlic cloves, finely chopped	1 tablespoon Worcestershire sauce
2 tablespoons finely chopped onion	2 tablespoons red wine vinegar
1 teaspoon chili flakes	2½ tablespoons molasses
½ teaspoon corn oil	1 teaspoon mustard powder
2 tablespoons water	¼ teaspoon salt
	½ teaspoon Tabasco sauce

1. In a food processor, puree the tomatoes, and set aside.
2. In a 1½-quart saucepan, sauté the garlic, onion, and chili flakes in oil for 2 minutes.
3. Add the pureed tomatoes and remaining ingredients, and simmer for 15 minutes, uncovered.

Yield: Makes 2 cups

Each ¼-cup serving has approximately 32 calories, 0.7 g. protein, 0.4 g. total fat (0.3 g. unsaturated fat, 0.1 g. saturated fat), 7.1 g. carbohydrates, 0 mg. cholesterol, 0.9 g. fiber, 95 mg. sodium, 19 mg. calcium.

Exchanges per serving: 1¼ vegetable.

Spicy Salsa

Fresh and spicy, with the refreshing tang of lime and the bite of peppers, this sauce is wonderful with fish, chicken, tortillas, you name it.

2 cups fresh chopped tomatoes (about 1 pound)	2 tablespoons chopped fresh cilantro leaves (coriander)
1 3-inch jalapeño pepper, chopped	juice of 2 limes
¼ medium onion, chopped	¼ teaspoon salt
2 garlic cloves, chopped	1 teaspoon corn oil

1. In a bowl combine the tomatoes, jalapeño pepper, onion, garlic, and cilantro. Add the lime juice, salt, and oil, and mix well.

Yield: Makes 2½ cups

Each ⅓-cup serving has approximately 30 calories, 0.6 g. protein, 1.8 g. total fat (1.5 g. unsaturated fat, 0.3 g. saturated fat), 3.6 g. carbohydrates, 0 mg. cholesterol, 0.9 g. fiber, 110 mg. sodium, 7.6 mg. calcium.

Exchanges per serving: ⅓ fat, ½ vegetable.

Enchilada Sauce

A fresh, not-too-spicy tomato sauce for Chicken Enchiladas (page 177) and Seafood Enchiladas (page 157).

2½ cups fresh Italian plum tomatoes (about 2 pounds)	2 teaspoons fresh oregano or ½ teaspoon dried
1 small onion, finely chopped	4 teaspoons chili powder
2 large garlic cloves, finely chopped	¼ cup plain non-fat yogurt

1. Core and seed the tomatoes. Puree in a blender, adding ¼ cup of water, if necessary, or in a food processor without added water.

2. Sauté the onion and garlic in a non-stick 10-inch fry pan for 2 minutes. Add the oregano, chili powder, and pureed tomatoes, and simmer together over low heat, uncovered, for 10 minutes. Stir in the yogurt until smooth.

Yield: Makes 2⅔ cups

Each ⅓-cup serving has approximately 25 calories, 1.2 g. protein, 0.4 g. total fat (0.3 g. unsaturated fat, 0.1 g. saturated fat), 5 g. carbohydrates, 0.1 mg. cholesterol, 1.5 g. fiber, 23 mg. sodium, 29 mg. calcium.

Exchanges per serving: 1 vegetable.

Green Tomatillo Sauce

This is a pungent, mildly spicy, and slightly chunky sauce made with tomatillos. Sometimes called *tomates verdes*, they are small green Mexican tomatoes with a light papery skin, about the size of cherry tomatoes, and are available where Spanish foods are sold.

1 pound tomatillos	1 tablespoon chopped onion
½ hot green jalapeño or cayenne chili pepper, finely chopped	½ cup chopped cilantro
2 large garlic cloves, finely chopped	¼ teaspoon salt

1. Remove the papery husk from each tomatillo. In a pot bring 1 quart of water to a simmer, and cook the tomatillos for 5 minutes. Drain the tomatillos through a colander.

2. In a blender or food processor puree the tomatillos, then add the pepper, garlic, onion, cilantro, and salt, and puree for 1 minute.

Yield: Makes 2 cups
Each ½-cup serving has approximately 30 calories, 1.4 g. protein, 0.3 g. total fat (0.1 g. unsaturated fat, 0 g. saturated fat), 6.7 g. carbohydrates, 0 mg. cholesterol, 2 g. fiber, 144 mg. sodium, 16 mg. calcium.
Exchanges per serving: 1 vegetable.

Wasabi

Hot, hot, hot. Serve this condiment with oriental dishes like California Nori Rolls (page 81) or Futomaki (page 79). Wasabi powder can be purchased in Chinese and oriental markets or the oriental section of supermarkets.

4   teaspoons wasabi powder
4   teaspoons water

1. In a small serving bowl mix the ingredients together until a thick paste forms.

Yield: Makes 4 teaspoons
One teaspoon serving has approximately 15 calories, 0.8 g. protein, 1 g. total fat (0.6 g. unsaturated fat, 0.2 g. saturated fat), 1.2 g. carbohydrates, 0 mg. cholesterol, 0.2 g. fiber, 0 mg. sodium, 18 mg. calcium.
Exchanges per serving: ⅕ starch.

Spicy Lemon Dipping Sauce

A zesty citrus sauce for fish and chicken that's great hot or cold.

½ tablespoon sugar
¼ cup hot water
2 garlic cloves

½ tablespoon jalapeño peppers
4 tablespoons fresh lemon juice
¼ teaspoon salt

1. Dissolve the sugar in the hot water.
2. Puree the garlic and jalapeño peppers in a food processor. Add the lemon juice, salt, and the sugar water, and mix well.

Yield: Makes ½ cup

One tablespoon has approximately 12 calories, 0.2 g. protein, 0 g. total fat (0 g. unsaturated fat, 0 g. saturated fat), 3.4 g. carbohydrates, 0 mg. cholesterol, 0.1 g. fiber, 149 mg. sodium, 5 mg. calcium.
Exchanges per serving: ⅙ starch.

Pesto Genovese

The traditional pesto, full of the fresh flavor of basil. Keep some in the freezer for quick pasta meals.

1 cup basil leaves, packed
1 clove garlic
1 tablespoon olive oil
½ tablespoon water

¼ teaspoon salt
1 tablespoon grated Parmesan
   cheese

1. Combine all the ingredients in a food processor and puree until smooth.

Yield: Makes about ½ cup

Each 2-tablespoon serving has approximately 48 calories, 1.2 g. protein, 4 g. total fat (3 g. unsaturated fat, 0.7 g. saturated fat), 3 g. carbohydrates, 1 mg. cholesterol, 1 g. fiber, 159 mg. sodium, 115 mg. calcium.
Exchanges per serving: ⅔ fat, ½ vegetable.

Peppery Mushroom Sauce

Serve with baked chicken, Veal Loaf (page 194), or practically any other beef or veal dish.

¾ pound sliced fresh mushrooms
1 tablespoon low-sodium soy sauce
¾ cup cold unsalted fat-free chicken or beef stock

1 tablespoon cornstarch
½ teaspoon freshly ground black pepper

1. Sauté the mushrooms in a 10-inch sauté pan for 5 minutes. Add the soy sauce and ½ cup of the stock, and cook for 2–3 minutes.
2. Mix the cornstarch with the remaining ¼ cup stock until lump-free. Add to the hot mushroom broth, and stir as sauce thickens. Season with black pepper.

Yield: Makes 1½ cups

Each ⅓-cup serving has approximately 32 calories, 2.1 g. protein, 0.4 g. total fat (0.2 g. unsaturated fat, 0.1 g. saturated fat), 6.3 g. carbohydrates, 0 mg. cholesterol, 1.6 g. fiber, 154 mg. sodium, 92 mg. calcium.
Exchanges per serving: 1¼ vegetable.

Tartar Sauce

A crunchy and creamy sauce for broiled fish or Three-Herb Crab Cakes (page 146).

1½ tablespoons reduced-calorie mayonnaise

2 tablespoons plain non-fat yogurt
1 teaspoon sweet relish

1. Combine the ingredients well in a small bowl.

Yield: Makes ¼ cup

One tablespoon has approximately 24 calories, 0.4 g. protein, 2 g. total fat (1.5 g. unsaturated fat, 0.4 g. saturated fat), 1.4 g. carbohydrates, 2 mg. cholesterol, 0 g. fiber, 57.4 mg. sodium, 14.4 mg. calcium.
Exchanges per serving: ½ fat.

Tomato Anchovy Sauce

The anchovies add a subtle kick to this rich, lightly peppery sauce. It's great on pasta and fish.

3 garlic cloves, minced
½ cup chopped onion
5 ounces fresh spinach (2½ cups packed)
½ tablespoon corn oil

1 can (2-ounce) anchovies, drained and finely chopped
1 can (28-ounce) crushed tomatoes
¼ teaspoon red pepper flakes

1. In a 2-quart saucepan sauté the garlic, onion, and spinach with the corn oil until the onions and spinach wilt, about 5 minutes.
2. Add the anchovies, tomatoes, and pepper flakes. Cook on medium-low heat for 15 minutes, covered, stirring occasionally.

Yield: Makes 3 cups
Each ¾-cup serving has approximately 90 calories, 6.1 g. protein, 3 g. total fat (2.1 g. unsaturated fat, 0.5 g. saturated fat), 13 g. carbohydrates, 10 mg. cholesterol, 4.5 g. fiber, 60 mg. sodium, 78 mg. calcium. Exchanges per serving: ½ fat, ½ meat, 2 vegetable.

Sweet and Sour Tomato Sauce

A mélange of sweet and sour tastes, plus a hint of ginger that is excellent with Spicy Cocktail Balls (page 77), as well as chicken and tongue.

2 teaspoons ginger, finely minced
2 garlic cloves, minced
1 medium onion, finely chopped
1 teaspoon corn oil
1⅓ pounds fresh Italian plum tomatoes
1 cup water

1 can (8-ounce) crushed pineapple
3 tablespoons red wine vinegar
½ teaspoon freshly ground black pepper
2 tablespoons brown sugar
2 teaspoons Worcestershire sauce

1. In a 2-quart pot sauté the ginger, garlic, and onion in the oil for 2 minutes.

2. Meanwhile, core and seed the tomatoes, and puree in a food processor.

3. Add the tomatoes, water, pineapple, vinegar, black pepper, sugar, and Worcestershire sauce, and cook over medium-low heat for 10 minutes, uncovered.

Yield: Makes 4 cups

Each ½-cup serving has approximately 52 calories, 0.8 g. protein, 0.7 g. total fat (0.6 g. unsaturated fat, 0.1 g. saturated fat), 12 g. carbohydrates, 0 mg. cholesterol, 1.2 g. fiber, 20 mg. sodium, 17 mg. calcium.
Exchanges per serving: 2 vegetable.

Creamy Tomato Sauce

A rich and creamy-tasting pink sauce for fish, chicken, or pasta.

2 or 3 Italian plum tomatoes to yield ½ cup puree	1 cup skim milk
1 tablespoon finely chopped shallots	⅛ teaspoon salt
1 tablespoon dry sherry	⅛ teaspoon white pepper
1 tablespoon margarine	1 teaspoon fresh marjoram, thyme, or rosemary
1 tablespoon unbleached flour	

1. Core and seed the tomatoes, then puree in a blender or food processor. You will need ½ cup of puree. Set aside.

2. In a heavy non-stick 8- or 10-inch sauté pan, cook the shallots with the sherry for 1–2 minutes, until translucent. Add the margarine, and when it has melted, sprinkle in the flour and stir to break up lumps. Slowly add the milk, stirring constantly to smooth any remaining lumps while the sauce thickens.

3. Add the tomato puree, salt, pepper, and herbs, and continue to cook for 2–3 minutes.

Yield: Makes 1⅓ cups

Each ⅓-cup serving has approximately 73 calories, 3 g. protein, 3.1 g. total fat (2.3 g. unsaturated fat, 0.7 g. saturated fat), 7.7 g. carbohydrates, 1 mg. cholesterol, 1 g. fiber, 137 mg. sodium, 85 mg. calcium.
Exchanges per serving: ½ fat, ¼ milk, ⅙ starch, ½ vegetable.

Italian Spaghetti Sauce with Fresh Herbs

Fresh tomatoes, fresh mushrooms, fresh herbs in a traditional sauce.

3 garlic cloves, finely chopped
1 medium onion, finely chopped
½ tablespoon olive oil
½ pound mushrooms, sliced
1 tablespoon dry red wine
2¾ pounds fresh Italian plum tomatoes, cored and cut into eighths, or 1 can (30-ounce) crushed Italian plum tomatoes plus 1 can (8-ounce) tomato sauce

1½ teaspoons crushed red pepper
½ teaspoon fresh oregano or ¼ teaspoon dried
2 tablespoons lightly chopped fresh basil
1 teaspoon chopped fresh marjoram
½ teaspoon salt

1. In a heavy 2-quart saucepan sauté the garlic and onion in the oil for 2–3 minutes, until the onions become soft and translucent. Add the mushrooms and wine, and cook for 5 minutes over low heat.

2. Meanwhile, in a blender or food processor puree the tomatoes with ¼ cup of water until smooth. You should have about 3½ cups of pureed tomatoes.

3. Add the tomatoes to the saucepan and simmer for 15 minutes over low heat. Add the red pepper, oregano, basil, marjoram, and salt, and cook for 5 more minutes.

Yield: Makes 5 cups

Each ⅔-cup serving has approximately 54 calories, 2.3 g. protein, 1.4 g. total fat (1 g. unsaturated fat, 0.2 g. saturated fat), 10 g. carbohydrates, 0 mg. cholesterol, 3.2 g. fiber, 148 mg. sodium, 33 mg. calcium.

Exchanges per serving: 2 vegetable.

Lemon Sauce

A tart, spicy, and slightly thick sauce for Steamed Spinach Dumplings (page 65), and Tuna with Cilantro Pesto (page 158).

¼ cup lemon juice
2 tablespoons unsalted fat-free chicken stock
1 tablespoon apple juice concentrate
1 tablespoon low-sodium soy sauce

2 teaspoons lemon peel
¼ teaspoon hot chili pepper
1½ teaspoons cornstarch
1 tablespoon cold water

1. Combine the lemon juice, chicken stock, apple juice, soy sauce, lemon peel, and chili pepper in a small pot and simmer for 1 minute.

2. In a separate bowl, combine the cornstarch with cold water, and stir until smooth. Add the cornstarch to the sauce, stirring as the mixture thickens.

Yield: Makes ½ cup

Each 2-tablespoon serving has approximately 18 calories, 0.4 g. protein, 0.1 g. total fat (0.1 g. unsaturated fat, 0 g. saturated fat), 4.6 g. carbohydrates, 0 mg. cholesterol, 0.1 g. fiber, 151 mg. sodium, 7 mg. calcium.

Exchanges per serving: ⅓ fruit.

Apple Rhubarb Sauce

Slightly tart and chunky sauce to serve with pork, chicken, and beef, and over frozen desserts.

2½ cups peeled and cubed Granny Smith apples (about 2 medium apples)
1⅓ cups fresh rhubarb stalks cut into 1-inch slices (about 2½ stalks)

1 or 2 packets non-nutritive sweetener (optional)

1. In a 1½-quart saucepan with a tight-fitting lid, combine the apples and rhubarb with ⅓ cup of water. Cook on low heat, covered, for 12–15 minutes. Taste for sweetness.

To microwave:

Combine the apples and rhubarb in a glass bowl. Cover tightly with plastic wrap and cook on high for 6 minutes.

Remove the plastic wrap. Lightly mash the mixture with the back of a spoon. Taste for sweetness, then recover with plastic wrap, and cook on high for 1 more minute.

Yield: Makes 4 cups

Each ¼-cup serving has approximately 25 calories, 0.3 g. protein, 0.2 g. total fat (0.1 g. unsaturated fat, 0 g. saturated fat), 6 g. carbohydrates, 0 mg. cholesterol, 1.3 g. fiber, 1.1 mg. sodium, 30 mg. calcium. Exchanges per serving: ½ fruit.

Cranberry Ginger Sauce

A tart side dish for chicken and meat.

3	cups cranberries	4	tablespoons dry marsala wine
1½	cups water	4	tablespoons sugar
1½	teaspoons ginger		

1. In a large saucepan combine all the ingredients, and boil for 5 minutes. Puree the mixture in a food processor.

Yield: Makes 2 cups

Each ¼-cup serving has approximately 48 calories, 0.2 g. protein, 0.1 g. total fat (0.05 g. unsaturated fat, 0 g. saturated fat), 11 g. carbohydrates, 0 mg. cholesterol, 1.5 g. fiber, 1 mg. sodium, 3.8 mg. calcium.
Exchanges per serving: ½ starch.

Mango Cream Sauce

A slightly tart and refreshing sauce for plain yogurt, poached chicken, and fresh fruits.

1 large ripe mango
2 tablespoons lime juice
2 tablespoons plain non-fat yogurt

1 teaspoon finely chopped fresh ginger

1. Cut the mango in half and scoop out the flesh with a spoon. You will need 1 cup of mango pulp for this recipe.
2. In a blender or food processor combine the mango pulp with the remaining ingredients, and puree for 1 minute.

Yield: Makes 1 cup

Each ¼-cup serving has approximately 39 calories, 0.6 g. protein, 0.2 g. total fat (0.1 g. unsaturated fat, 0 g. saturated fat), 10 g. carbohydrates, 0.1 mg. cholesterol, 2 g. fiber, 6 mg. sodium, 20 mg. calcium. Exchanges per serving: ½ fruit.

Raspberry Sauce

A lovely light berry sauce that complements a variety of dishes— fresh peaches, poached pears, frozen yogurt, or a Chocolate Meringue Cake (page 281), for instance.

2 packages (12-ounce size) unsweetened frozen raspberries, defrosted

1 tablespoon chopped fresh lemon mint

1. Puree the raspberries in a food processor until smooth, then stir in the lemon mint.

Yield: Makes 2½ cups

Each ¼-cup serving has approximately 37.4 calories, 0.7 g. protein, 0.7 g. total fat (0.7 g. unsaturated fat, 0 g. saturated fat), 9.5 g. carbohydrates, 0 mg. cholesterol, 2.6 g. fiber, 0 mg. sodium, 0 mg. calcium. Exchanges per serving: ⅔ fruit.

Bittersweet Chocolate Cherry Sauce

Serve with frozen yogurt, ice milk, Chocolate Meringue Cake (page 281), over fresh fruit, or Chocolate Cake (page 278).

2 cups canned sugar-free cherries	4 packets non-nutritive sweet-
2 teaspoons cornstarch	ener
¼ cup water	
2 tablespoons unsweetened cocoa powder	

1. Drain the cherries, reserving the juice separately.
2. In a small bowl combine the cornstarch and water until smooth.
3. In a small saucepan combine the cherry juice and cocoa. Stir together over low heat until the cocoa dissolves. Add the cornstarch mixture and the cherries, and stir over low heat as mixture thickens.

To microwave, whisk together the cherry juice and cocoa in a microwave-safe bowl until smooth, and cook for 1 minute on high. Stir in the cherries and cornstarch, and cook for 1 minute on high, stir, cook for another minute, stir, and cook for 1 more minute, until the mixture has slightly thickened. Stir in the non-nutritive sweetener.

Yield: Makes 2 cups

Each ¼-cup serving has approximately 66 calories, 1 g. protein, 3 g. total fat (0.1 g. unsaturated fat, 0.2 g. saturated fat), 16.2 g. carbohydrates, 0 mg. cholesterol, 1 g. fiber, 1 mg. sodium, 9.7 mg. calcium. Exchanges per serving: 1 fruit.

Mocha Sauce

A smooth sauce for frozen desserts and fresh fruit.

6 tablespoons unsweetened cocoa powder	2½ tablespoons instant coffee
1 cup skim milk	6 packets non-nutritive sweetener

1. In a saucepan combine the cocoa powder and skim milk over low heat, stirring constantly with a whisk until the cocoa is well dissolved. Stir in the instant coffee and non-nutritive sweetener.

Yield: Makes 1 cup

Each 2-tablespoon serving has approximately 25 calories, 1.8 g. protein, 0.8 g. total fat (0.3 g. unsaturated fat, 0.5 g. saturated fat), 4.7 g. carbohydrates, 0.5 mg. cholesterol, 1.2 g. fiber, 17 mg. sodium, 45 mg. calcium.

Exchanges per serving: ⅓ milk.

Fish and Seafood

Poached Fish with Julienne
  Vegetables
Fish Fillets with Red Pepper
  Glaze
Broiled Fillets with Fresh
  Sweet Peppers and Mint
Bluefish with Spicy Salsa
Cajun Catfish
Three-Herb Crab Cakes
Flounder Stuffed with
  Crabmeat and Basil
Mako in Mustard Curry Sauce
Steamed Mussels in Herb
  Broth
Orange Roughy with Apricot
  Glaze
Salmon Wrapped in Phyllo
Poached Salmon with
  Horseradish-Caper Sauce
Pan-Broiled Teriyaki Salmon

Scallops in Black Bean Sauce
Sautéed Scallops with
  Chopped Tomato, Garlic,
  and Herbs
Spicy Stir-Fried Scallops with
  Asparagus
Seafood Brochettes with
  Rosemary
Seafood Newburg with
  Asparagus
Seafood Enchiladas
Chinese Sweet and Sour Sea
  Trout
Tuna with Cilantro Pesto
Baked Tuna Niçoise
Shrimp with Feta Cheese
Zuppa di Pesce
Ceviche with Chunky
  Vegetable Salsa

Poached Fish with Julienne Vegetables

Crunchy fresh vegetables and a hint of ginger distinguish this delicate dish, which you can make with your favorite fish.

3 cups Basic Fish Stock (page 100) or vegetable stock	1 medium carrot, peeled and cut into 2-inch julienne strips
½ teaspoon salt	1 small zucchini, cut into 2-inch julienne strips
1 pound fish fillets (catfish, sole, flounder, perch, or salmon)	1 small red bell pepper, cut into 2-inch julienne strips
1 tablespoon finely sliced fresh ginger	1 lemon, quartered

1. In a 10-inch fry pan, heat the stock and salt to a simmer. Reduce to lowest heat possible; the stock should not bubble at all.

2. Lay the fillets in one layer in the pot, cover with ginger slices and vegetable strips, and poach for 8 minutes.

3. With a slotted spatula, carefully transfer the fish fillets and vegetables to individual warmed serving plates, and garnish each with a lemon wedge.

Yield: Serves 4

Each serving has approximately 149 calories, 21.3 g. protein, 5 g. total fat (3.1 g. unsaturated fat, 1.1 g. saturated fat), 4 g. carbohydrates, 65.8 mg. cholesterol, 1.2 g. fiber, 79 mg. sodium, 56 mg. calcium. Exchanges per serving: 2½ meat, ½ vegetable.

Fish Fillets with Red Pepper Glaze

These fish fillets have a sweet caramelized taste that's faintly oriental. We offer a choice of fish and a choice of garnish. We like it with Wild and Brown Rice (page 231).

⅔ pound red bell peppers, cored and seeds removed	½ tablespoon cornstarch
1 tablespoon toasted sesame oil	1 tablespoon cold water
½ teaspoon crushed hot pepper flakes	1 pound fish fillets (orange roughy, perch, catfish)
1 tablespoon granulated sugar	2 tablespoons fresh sliced scallions or chopped cilantro
¼ teaspoon salt	

1. Preheat broiler and broiler pan.
2. Blanch the red pepper in 2 cups of boiling water for 1 minute, then puree in a food processor. Add the sesame oil, hot pepper flakes, sugar, and salt, and mix the glaze well.
3. In a bowl mix the cornstarch and water to a paste, then add the glaze and stir until thickened.
4. Brush the fish on both sides with the glaze, and transfer to the heated broiling pan. Broil the fish for 5 minutes on one side only.
5. Serve garnished with scallions or cilantro.

Yield: Serves 4

Each serving has approximately 172 calories, 22 g. protein, 5.6 g. total fat (4.2 g. unsaturated fat, 0.8 g. saturated fat), 8 g. carbohydrates, 47.6 mg. cholesterol, 1.3 g. fiber, 221 mg. sodium, 128 mg. calcium. Exchanges per serving: 3 meat, ½ vegetable.

Broiled Fillets with Fresh Sweet Peppers and Mint

Colorful vegetables add crunch and sweetness to the delicate fish; mint is a refreshing surprise.

½ red onion, peeled and thinly sliced	2 teaspoons corn oil
	½ teaspoon salt
1 medium red bell pepper, seeded, and cut into strips	1 pound fresh fish fillets (perch, flounder, catfish, scrod)
1 medium yellow bell pepper, seeded, and cut into strips	¼ teaspoon freshly ground white or black pepper
2 garlic cloves, finely chopped	1 tablespoon fresh lemon juice
½ tablespoon Worcestershire sauce	4 sprigs fresh mint
1 tablespoon water	
2 tablespoons chopped fresh mint or ½ tablespoon dried mint	

1. Preheat broiler and broiling pan.
2. In an 8-inch, non-stick sauté pan, cook the onion, pepper strips, and garlic with the Worcestershire sauce and water over medium heat until the vegetables soften, about 4–5 minutes. Add the mint, oil, and

¼ teaspoon of the salt. Cook for 1 more minute, then remove from heat and set aside.

3. Lay the fish on the broiling pan. Sprinkle the pepper over the fish, together with the remaining ¼ teaspoon salt and the lemon juice. Broil the fish for 5 minutes on one side only. Spoon the cooked vegetables over the fish, and broil for 3 more minutes.

4. Serve on individual warmed dinner plates and garnish each with a sprig of fresh mint.

Yield: Serves 4

Each serving has approximately 171 calories, 21.3 g. protein, 7.3 g. total fat (5 g. unsaturated fat, 1.4 g. saturated fat), 4.3 g. carbohydrates, 66 mg. cholesterol, 1 g. fiber, 361 mg. sodium, 60 mg. calcium. Exchanges per serving: 3 meat, 1 vegetable.

Bluefish with Spicy Salsa

Fresh and spicy, with the refreshing tang of lime and the bite of peppers. You can cook this in the oven or microwave, and use this sauce to spice up any fish.

1   **pound bluefish**
2½ **cups Spicy Salsa (page 129)**

1. If baking in the oven, preheat oven to 425° F.

2. For oven baking, lay the fish in a baking dish and bake, uncovered, for 8 minutes. Spoon the salsa over the fish, and bake for 4 more minutes.

For microwave, place the fish in a microwave-safe baking dish, cover tightly with plastic wrap, and cook on medium-high power for 3 minutes, rotating the dish after 1½ minutes. Uncover, spoon the salsa over the fish, recover the dish tightly, and cook on medium-high power for 2 minutes.

Yield: Serves 4

Each serving has approximately 180 calories, 24 g. protein, 6.2 g. total fat (4.3 g. unsaturated fat, 1.3 g. saturated fat), 7.3 g. carbohydrates, 67 mg. cholesterol, 1.7 g. fiber, 287 mg. sodium, 23 mg. calcium. Exchanges per serving: 3 meat, ½ vegetable.

Cajun Catfish

Hot and spicy — just what you'd expect from Cajun-style cooking.

4 4-ounce catfish fillets	¼ teaspoon garlic powder
1 ounce sugar-free wheat flakes cereal (like NutriGrain), finely ground (¼ cup ground)	½ teaspoon cayenne pepper
	½ teaspoon black pepper
	½ teaspoon white pepper
1 tablespoon paprika	½ teaspoon thyme
¼ teaspoon salt	1 tablespoon oil
¼ teaspoon onion powder	

1. Wash the fish fillets and pat dry.
2. In a bowl mix the ground wheat flakes and all the seasonings. Pour the dry mixture onto a piece of foil or wax paper, and dip the fillets into the seasoning, coating both sides.
3. In a heavy cast-iron fry pan heat the oil. Fry the fillets for 2 minutes on each side. Lay the fillets on a plate lined with a paper towel, cover with another paper towel, and pat to remove excess oil.

Yield: Serves 4

Each serving has approximately 170 calories, 21 g. protein, 8.5 g. total fat (6 g. unsaturated fat, 1.6 g. saturated fat), 1.8 g. carbohydrates, 66 mg. cholesterol, 0.6 g. fiber, 206 mg. sodium, 56 mg. calcium. Exchanges per serving: ¼ fat, 3 meat.

Three-Herb Crab Cakes

Tarragon, dill, and basil, mixed with fresh bread crumbs, add extra flavor to tender crabmeat. Top with Tartar Sauce (page 133).

1 pound fresh backfin crabmeat	1 teaspoon chopped fresh tarragon
1 celery stalk, finely chopped	
¼ teaspoon paprika	1 teaspoon chopped fresh dill
2 tablespoons reduced-calorie mayonnaise	1 teaspoon chopped fresh basil
	2 tablespoons finely ground fresh bread crumbs
⅛ teaspoon ground white pepper	

1. Preheat broiler.
2. Combine all the ingredients and mold into 4 patties. Lay them on a baking pan.

3. Broil for 5 minutes on each side. Carefully remove from the pan and serve on warmed plates.

Yield: Makes 4 good-sized crab cakes

Each serving has approximately 155 calories, 23.4 g. protein, 4.7 g. total fat (3.2 g. unsaturated fat, 1 g. saturated fat), 3.1 g. carbohydrates, 116 mg. cholesterol, 0.3 g. fiber, 405 mg. sodium, 125 mg. calcium.

Exchanges per serving: 3 meat.

Flounder Stuffed with Crabmeat and Basil

A creamy, aromatic basil mixture and chewy crabmeat encased in lightly breaded fillets. Serve alone or with Peppery Mushroom Sauce (page 133) or Lemon Sauce (page 137).

4 flounder fillets, about ¾ pound total	1 tablespoon reduced-calorie mayonnaise
¼ cup bread crumbs	⅛ teaspoon salt
½ cup basil leaves, packed	¼ pound crabmeat
1 small garlic clove	⅛ teaspoon paprika

1. Preheat oven to 425° F.
2. Wash the flounder fillets and pat dry with paper towel. Coat with breadcrumbs and set aside.
3. In the food processor combine and puree together the basil, garlic, mayonnaise, and salt. Transfer to a bowl and stir in the crabmeat.
4. Spoon 2 tablespoons of basil-crabmeat filling on each fillet, then roll the fish over the filling to create open-sided roulades.
5. Lay the flounder rolls on a bake-and-serve casserole, sprinkle lightly with paprika, and bake for 8 minutes.

Yield: Serves 4

Each serving has approximately 146 calories, 22.5 g. protein, 3.1 g. total fat (2 g. unsaturated fat, 0.6 g. saturated fat), 5.8 g. carbohydrates, 70 mg. cholesterol, 0.5 g. fiber, 289 mg. sodium, 78 mg. calcium.

Exchanges per serving: 3 meat.

Mako in Mustard Curry Sauce

Mako is shark, a tender, meaty, and chewy fish that tastes somewhat like swordfish. Here it's marinated and baked in a spicy, tart sauce.

1 cup plain non-fat yogurt	1½ teaspoons curry powder
3 tablespoons stone-ground mustard	4 teaspoons chutney
1 tablespoon horseradish	4 4-ounce shark steaks

1. In a bowl whisk together the yogurt, mustard, horseradish, curry powder, and chutney, and pour it into a non-aluminum bake-and-serve dish just big enough to hold the fish in one layer, about 9 inches square.
2. Lay fish steaks in the marinade, coating them well. Marinate for 6 hours in the refrigerator.
3. Preheat oven to 425° F.
4. Bake the fish for 8 minutes.
5. Spoon the sauce from the bottom of the pan over the fish steaks, and serve.

Yield: Serves 4

Each serving has approximately 183 calories, 26 g. protein, 5.3 g. total fat (3.4 g. unsaturated fat, 1.3 g. saturated fat), 7 g. carbohydrates, 45 mg. cholesterol, 0.4 g. fiber, 295 mg. sodium, 134 mg. calcium. Exchanges per serving: 3 meat, ⅓ milk.

Steamed Mussels in Herb Broth

Mussels in a rich fish broth flavored with three herbs.

2 dozen small fresh mussels	6 tablespoons dry white wine
4 large garlic cloves, finely chopped	¾ teaspoon freshly ground black pepper
1 small onion, finely chopped	¼ teaspoon salt
1 tablespoon olive oil	½ cup chopped fresh basil
3 cups fresh Basic Fish Stock (page 100)	2 teaspoons fresh marjoram
	5 sprigs fresh thyme

1. Soak the mussels in cold water for 5 minutes, then drain. Only use closed mussels.

2. In a non-aluminum 3-quart pot or saucepan sauté the garlic and onion in the oil for 1 minute, until the onions are translucent. Add the stock and wine, and bring to a simmer. Add the pepper, salt, basil, marjoram, thyme, and the clean mussels, cover the pot, and cook for 3 minutes over medium-low heat. All mussel shells should open; if many are not, recover the pot and cook for 1 more minute. Discard any mussels that have still not opened.

3. Serve each person a bowl with 6 mussels and a portion of the herbed broth.

Yield: Serves 4

Each serving has approximately 105 calories, 4.4 g. protein, 11.5 g. total fat (5.3 g. unsaturated fat, 0.9 g. saturated fat), 6.1 g. carbohydrates, 18.8 mg. cholesterol, 2.3 g. fiber, 219 mg. sodium, 95 mg. calcium.
Exchanges per serving: ¾ fat, ⅔ meat, ¼ starch, 1 vegetable.

Orange Roughy with Apricot Glaze

A sweet fish under a sweet, caramelized glaze with a tang of mustard.

2 teaspoons margarine, melted	4 4-ounce fillets of orange
4 tablespoons orange or apricot	roughy or other firm fish
low-sugar marmalade	
2 teaspoons stone-ground	
mustard	

1. Preheat broiler and a 9 × 9-inch baking pan.

2. Melt the margarine in a saucepan, remove from heat, and stir in the marmalade and mustard to form a glaze.

3. Place the fish in the preheated pan, and top with half the glaze. Broil for 5 minutes, then brush on the remaining glaze and broil for 3 more minutes on the same side.

Yield: Serves 4

Each serving has approximately 174 calories, 20.7 g. protein, 6.8 g. total fat (4.5 g. unsaturated fat, 1.5 g. saturated fat), 6.1 g. carbohydrates, 65.8 mg. cholesterol, 0 g. fiber, 110 mg. sodium, 47.2 mg. calcium.
Exchanges per serving: 3 meat, ¼ starch.

Salmon Wrapped in Phyllo

Moist salmon and grainy mustard wrapped in flaky phyllo dough.

10 ounces fresh or defrosted frozen spinach	easier to work with than frozen sheets, readily available in supermarkets)
1½ tablespoons margarine	
8 sheets phyllo dough (if possible, buy fresh phyllo at gourmet stores or Middle Eastern markets, because it's	4 4-ounce salmon fillets, skin removed
	4 teaspoons stone-ground mustard

1. Preheat oven to 425° F.

2. Steam the spinach for 5 minutes, or sauté it for 4 minutes, or microwave it for 3 minutes on high, until tender. Drain the spinach and let it cool, then squeeze out all excess water so it is virtually dry. Set aside.

3. Melt the margarine in a small saucepan.

4. Lay 2 sheets of phyllo dough horizontally on a dry countertop, and wrap the remaining sheets tightly in plastic to prevent their drying out. Using a pastry brush, lightly brush the right half of the phyllo sheet with a little margarine, and fold it over the left half, making a rectangle about 12 × 8 inches. Lightly brush the dough with a little margarine.

5. Lay a salmon fillet in the center of the phyllo. Spread 1 teaspoon of mustard on the salmon, then spoon on ¼ of the spinach. Fold the top and bottom sides of the phyllo over the salmon, then fold in the two sides, forming a neat packet encasing the salmon. Brush all sides of the packet lightly with margarine, and place it on a cookie sheet. Repeat this procedure for the remaining 3 salmon fillets.

6. Bake for 8–10 minutes, until the phyllo begins to brown. If you don't bake the packets immediately, cover them with a cloth towel so the phyllo doesn't dry out.

Yield: Serves 4

Each serving has approximately 259 calories, 26.8 g. protein, 9.5 g. total fat (6.1 g. unsaturated fat, 1.5 g. saturated fat), 17 g. carbohydrates, 59 mg. cholesterol, 2.4 g. fiber, 338 mg. sodium, 121 mg. calcium.

Exchanges per serving: 3 meat, 1 starch, ½ vegetable.

Poached Salmon with Horseradish-Caper Sauce

Tender salmon with a tart and pungent creamy sauce.

2 tablespoons reduced-calorie mayonnaise	4 cups Basic Fish Stock (page 100)
2 tablespoons plain, non-fat yogurt	½ cup white wine
	4 4-ounce salmon fillets
2 tablespoons capers	½ teaspoon freshly ground pepper
2 tablespoons prepared horse-radish	4 fresh lettuce leaves
	1 lemon, quartered

1. In a small bowl combine the mayonnaise, yogurt, capers, and horseradish. Set aside.

2. In a saucepan large enough to hold the fish in one layer, combine the fish stock and wine. (There should be enough liquid to slightly cover the fish; add water if more liquid is necessary.) Bring the liquid to a simmer, turn heat to very low so that no bubbles are visible, add the salmon, and poach for 10 minutes.

3. Remove the fish from the pot carefully with a slotted spatula, and lay each fillet on an individual warmed dinner plate. Sprinkle some pepper over each fillet. Garnish each plate with a lettuce leaf filled with 2 tablespoons of the horseradish sauce and a wedge of lemon.

Yield: Serves 4

Each serving has approximately 197 calories, 23 g. protein, 9.7 g. total fat (7.1 g. unsaturated fat, 1.6 g. saturated fat), 1.8 g. carbohydrates, 65 mg. cholesterol, 0.1 g. fiber, 221 mg. sodium, 33 mg. calcium. Exchanges per serving: ½ fat, 3 meat.

Pan-Broiled Teriyaki Salmon

Quick and easy salmon with a rich soy flavor.

½ tablespoon toasted sesame oil
2 tablespoons mirin (sweet rice wine, available in oriental and gourmet markets)

2 tablespoons low-sodium soy sauce
4 4-ounce fresh salmon fillets, skinned
2 scallions, finely chopped

1. In a 10-inch sauté pan, heat the sesame oil, mirin, and soy sauce.
2. Add the salmon fillets, and pan-fry for 2 minutes over medium heat. Carefully turn the fish over with a spatula and cook for 2 more minutes, or until the salmon is pink on the outside and barely pink inside.
3. Garnish with chopped scallions and serve on heated plates.

Yield: Serves 4

Each serving has approximately 162 calories, 23 g. protein, 5.4 g. total fat (3.7 g. unsaturated fat, 1 g. saturated fat), 2 g. carbohydrates, 59 mg. cholesterol, 0.1 g. fiber, 393 mg. sodium, 59 mg. calcium. Exchanges per serving: 3 meat.

Scallops in Black Bean Sauce

Tender scallops, crisp vegetables, and pungent beans for an oriental flavor.

3 tablespoons fermented black beans (available in oriental and gourmet markets)
⅔ cup water
1 tablespoon sesame oil
2 garlic cloves, finely chopped

½ tablespoon fresh ginger, peeled and finely chopped
¼ teaspoon crushed red pepper
½ small red bell pepper, seeded, cored, and cut into strips
3 scallions, finely chopped
1 pound sea or bay scallops

1. Soak the black beans in the water for 15 minutes to remove excess salt. Rinse through a colander under a slow stream of water until the drained water is clear.
2. Heat the oil, garlic, ginger, and crushed red pepper in a wok or

10-inch sauté pan for 2 minutes. Add the bell pepper strips, scallions, and the scallops, and sauté until tender, about 3 minutes for sea scallops or 2 minutes for bay scallops. Add the rinsed black beans, and cook for 1 minute.

Yield: Serves 4

Each serving has approximately 189 calories, 13 g. protein, 6.2 g. total fat (3.6 g. unsaturated fat, 2.3 g. saturated fat), 6 g. carbohydrates, 21.4 mg. cholesterol, 3.1 g. fiber, 164 mg. sodium, 73 mg. calcium. Exchanges per serving: 3 meat.

Sautéed Scallops with Chopped Tomato, Garlic, and Herbs

Tender chewy scallops in a light herb sauce with a mild mustard tang. A quick refreshing summer dinner.

1 pound sea scallops	1 teaspoon fresh thyme or
¼ cup unbleached flour	½ teaspoon dried
1 tablespoon olive oil	1 tablespoon stone-ground
2 garlic cloves, finely chopped	mustard
¼ cup dry white wine	
3 medium plum tomatoes, seeded and chopped	

1. Rinse the scallops, drain in a fine-mesh strainer, and pat dry with paper towels.
2. Pour the flour on a piece of foil, dredge the scallops in it, and shake off excess flour.
3. In a 10-inch fry pan heat the oil over medium-low heat. Add the garlic, then the scallops, and sauté 2 minutes. Add the wine, a little at a time. Add the chopped tomato, thyme, and mustard, and cook for 1–2 minutes. Serve immediately.

Yield: Serves 4

Each serving has approximately 168 calories, 20.2 g. protein, 4.6 g. total fat (3.6 g. unsaturated fat, 0.4 g. saturated fat), 8.5 g. carbohydrates, 38 mg. cholesterol, 0.8 g. fiber, 235 mg. sodium, 39 mg. calcium.
Exchanges per serving: 3 meat, ¼ vegetable.

Spicy Stir-Fried Scallops with Asparagus

A tangy dish of vivid flavors that gets spicier by the mouthful. Serve it with rice or Chinese noodles.

1	tablespoon sesame or peanut oil
2	garlic cloves, finely chopped
½	tablespoon fresh grated ginger
1	teaspoon red pepper flakes
1	pound sea scallops
1⅓	pounds asparagus, white stalks removed and cut in 1-inch diagonal slices
3	scallions, cut in ¼-inch diagonal slices

Sauce:

1	tablespoon water
1	tablespoon low-sodium soy sauce
1	teaspoon cornstarch
1	tablespoon sherry
2	tablespoons sesame seeds

1. Heat the oil in a wok or 12-inch fry or sauté pan. Add the garlic, ginger, and red pepper flakes. Cook on medium heat for 2 minutes. Add the scallops and stir-fry for 2 minutes, or until they become firm. Remove the scallops to a plate.

2. Add the asparagus and scallions to the center of the pan, and stir-fry on medium heat until the asparagus is crisp-tender, about 3 to 4 minutes. If the pan gets too dry, add a few tablespoons of water.

3. In a small bowl combine 1 tablespoon of water with the soy sauce, cornstarch, and sherry. Stir to dissolve the cornstarch.

4. Return the scallops to the pan and push everything to one side. Add the cornstarch mixture to the center of the pan and heat until the sauce thickens, stirring frequently. If the sauce gets too thick, add enough water to bring it to the desired consistency. Then combine with the scallops and asparagus so the sauce coats them nicely. Sprinkle with sesame seeds.

Yield: Serves 4

Each serving has approximately 203 calories, 25 g. protein, 7 g. total fat (6 g. unsaturated fat, 1 g. saturated fat), 11 g. carbohydrates, 37.4 mg. cholesterol, 2.7 g. fiber, 337 mg. sodium, 115 mg. calcium. Exchanges per serving: 3 meat, 1½ vegetable.

Seafood Brochettes with Rosemary

Meaty chunks of fish and seafood basted in a citrus marinade and broiled until just tender.

⅓ pound 1-inch-thick tuna
steak, trimmed of skin
⅓ pound 1-inch-thick swordfish
steak, trimmed of skin
8 large shrimp
¼ pound sea scallops
4 10-inch skewers
1 tablespoon olive oil

1 teaspoon low-sodium soy
sauce
1 tablespoon chopped fresh
rosemary or 1 teaspoon dried
1½ tablespoons lemon juice
⅓ teaspoon coarsely ground
black pepper

1. Preheat the broiler, and set the broiler rack at the middle level.

2. Cut the tuna and swordfish steaks each into 8 cubes. Peel and devein the shrimp.

3. Take a skewer and thread it first with a piece of tuna, then a scallop, a shrimp, and a piece of swordfish, then a second piece of each fish in the same order. Thread the remaining 3 skewers in the same way. Place the skewers on a broiling pan.

4. In a bowl, combine the olive oil, soy sauce, rosemary, and lemon juice. Using a basting brush, baste the fish on one side with the liquid, then sprinkle with some pepper.

5. Broil (or barbecue) the fish for 3 minutes. Turn the skewers over, baste with the remaining liquid, sprinkle with more pepper, and broil for 2½ more minutes.

Yield: Serves 4

Each serving has approximately 174 calories, 27 g. protein, 6 g. total fat (3.2 g. unsaturated fat, 1.1 g. saturated fat), 1.8 g. carbohydrates, 84 mg. cholesterol, 0.1 g. fiber, 221 mg. sodium, 34 mg. calcium. Exchanges per serving: 3½ meat.

Seafood Newburg with Asparagus

A creamy saffron sauce over tender chunks of seafood. Excellent over rice or pasta.

4 teaspoons margarine	1 clove garlic, finely chopped
½ pound shrimp, peeled and deveined	2 tablespoons dry sherry
	1 tablespoon unbleached flour
¼ pound bay scallops	10 ounces skim milk
½ pound crabmeat, shredded	¼ teaspoon saffron
½ pound asparagus, trimmed of tough lower stalks	¼ teaspoon salt
	⅛ teaspoon white pepper
2 tablespoons chopped shallots	

1. In a 10-inch skillet melt 1 teaspoon of the margarine, add the shrimp and scallops, and, stirring frequently, sauté until the shrimp is pink, about 3–4 minutes. Add the crabmeat, remove from heat, and set aside.

2. Cut off the asparagus tips and slice the stalks into 1-inch pieces. Steam the asparagus tips and pieces for 4 minutes, or microwave, covered, for 3 minutes on high. Set aside.

3. In a 2-quart non-aluminum saucepan cook the shallots, garlic, and sherry together on medium heat for 1 minute. Add the remaining 3 teaspoons of margarine, let melt, then sprinkle with the flour and stir for 30 seconds to keep the mixture smooth. Add the milk, a little at a time, stirring constantly to avoid lumps. The sauce will thicken as it heats. Stir in the saffron, salt, and pepper, and reduce heat to low. Add the cooked seafood and asparagus, stir to coat them with the sauce, and cook for 2 more minutes.

Yield: Serves 4

Each serving has approximately 235 calories, 32.3 g. protein, 6.3 g. total fat (4.1 g. unsaturated fat, 1.2 g. saturated fat), 9.4 g. carbohydrates, 153 mg. cholesterol, 1 g. fiber, 504 mg. sodium, 202 mg. calcium.

Exchanges per serving: 3½ meat, ¼ milk, ⅕ starch, ½ vegetable.

Seafood Enchiladas

Three kinds of seafood in a slightly spicy sauce make a chewy enchilada filling.

2 garlic cloves, finely chopped	2 cups Enchilada Sauce (page
1 teaspoon corn oil	130) or Green Tomatillo Sauce
½ pound large shrimp, peeled	(page 130)
and deveined	8 6-inch prepared corn tortillas
6 ounces bay scallops	2 ounces grated part-skim
4 ounces crabmeat, shredded	mozzarella cheese

1. Preheat oven to 375° F.
2. Heat the garlic and oil in a 10-inch skillet, and cook on medium heat for 1 minute.
3. Cut each shrimp in half across its width, and add the shrimp halves and scallops. Sauté until the shrimp become pink and bay scallops rigid, about 2–3 minutes.
4. Stir in the crabmeat and ⅓ cup of the enchilada or green tomatillo sauce. Remove the mixture from heat, and set aside.
5. To soften the tortillas, steam or microwave them, two at a time, for 10 seconds.
6. Spread ⅔ cup of the sauce on the bottom of an 8 × 14-inch pan. Fill each tortilla with ¼ cup of the seafood, roll up to form a crepe, and lay seam side up on the sauce. Pour the remaining 1 cup of sauce over the tortillas, and sprinkle with the grated cheese. Bake for 15 minutes or microwave, covered, for 5 minutes on high.

Yield: Serves 8
Each serving has approximately 165 calories, 16.6 g. protein, 3.8 g. total fat (2.3 g. unsaturated fat, 1.1 g. saturated fat), 17 g. carbohydrates, 68.3 mg. cholesterol, 3.3 g. fiber, 212 mg. sodium, 130 mg. calcium.
Exchanges per serving: 2 meat, 1 starch, ½ vegetable.

Chinese Sweet and Sour Sea Trout

We use sea trout, but this sweet and sour sauce enlivens any light fish fillet, or even ½-inch-thick swordfish steaks.

1 tablespoon low-sodium soy sauce	1 tablespoon cornstarch
1 tablespoon sherry	2 tablespoons cold water
½ tablespoon vinegar	1 tablespoon corn oil
⅓ cup unsalted, fat-free chicken stock, fish stock, or water	2 garlic cloves, finely chopped
1 tablespoon sugar	4 4-ounce fillets of sea trout
	2 scallions, finely sliced

1. In a small saucepan combine the soy sauce, sherry, vinegar, and stock or water. Add the sugar, and stir to dissolve. Set aside.

2. In a small bowl mix the cornstarch and 2 tablespoons of cold water until lump-free. Set aside.

3. In a 10-inch skillet heat the oil over medium heat, add the garlic, and cook for 1 minute. Add the fish, and cook for 2 minutes on each side. Turn heat to low, and add the sweet and sour sauce and the cornstarch mixture, and simmer for 2 minutes. The sauce will thicken slightly. Spoon some of the sauce from the side of the pan onto the top of the fish fillets.

4. Serve the fillets topped with scallions.

Yield: Serves 4

Each serving has approximately 178 calories, 19.3 g. protein, 7.6 g. total fat (4.7 g. unsaturated fat, 1.6 g. saturated fat), 6 g. carbohydrates, 94 mg. cholesterol, 0.1 g. fiber, 217 mg. sodium, 28 mg. calcium.

Exchanges per serving: ¼ fat, 3 meat.

Tuna with Cilantro Pesto

The piquant flavor of cilantro on chewy tuna steaks you can bake or broil. Serve them with Lemon Sauce (page 137).

¾ cup cilantro (coriander), packed	1 teaspoon low-sodium soy sauce
1 large garlic clove	4 4-ounce tuna steaks, ¾ inch thick or less
2 teaspoons olive oil	

1. Preheat oven to 425° F. or preheat broiler and broiling pan.
2. Rinse the cilantro in cold water two or three times until the water is clean. Drain through a colander.
3. In a food processor combine the cilantro with the garlic, oil, and soy sauce, and puree to make cilantro pesto.
4. Bake or broil the fish for 8 minutes. During the last 2 minutes put 1 tablespoon of the cilantro pesto over each fish steak.

Yield: Serves 4

Each serving has approximately 159 calories, 22.7 g. protein, 6.9 g. total fat (4.7 g. unsaturated fat, 1.5 g. saturated fat), 0.5 g. carbohydrates, 44.2 mg. cholesterol, 0 g. fiber, 153 mg. sodium, 10 mg. calcium.
Exchanges per serving: 3 meat, ½ vegetable.

Baked Tuna Niçoise

The meaty taste of tuna under a bed of Mediterranean-style vegetables.

1 small onion, sliced into thin rings	2 tablespoons chopped fresh basil
2 garlic cloves, finely chopped	½ tablespoon capers
1 teaspoon olive oil	8 niçoise or gaeta olives (about 1 ounce)
½ large yellow bell pepper, cut into strips	¼ teaspoon freshly ground pepper
4 plum tomatoes, quartered	4 4-ounce fresh tuna steaks, 1 inch thick
1 tablespoon red wine vinegar or balsamic vinegar	

1. Preheat oven to 425° F.
2. In a 10-inch, non-stick sauté pan sauté the onion and garlic in the olive oil for 2–3 minutes.
3. Add the pepper strips, quartered tomatoes, and vinegar, and cook for 2 minutes. Add the basil, capers, and olives, and grind the pepper on top. Keep the mixture warm on very low heat while the fish cooks.
4. Lay the tuna steaks in a baking dish, and bake for 8–10 minutes, or until the inside is slightly pink.

5. Transfer the tuna steaks to heated serving plates and top with the warm vegetables niçoise.

Yield: Serves 4

Each serving has approximately 185 calories, 28.4 g. protein, 4 g. total fat (3 g. unsaturated fat, 0.7 g. saturated fat), 9.5 g. carbohydrates, 51 mg. cholesterol, 3 g. fiber, 132 mg. sodium, 69.3 mg. calcium. Exchanges per serving: 3 meat, 1 vegetable.

Shrimp with Feta Cheese

Shrimp in a creamy, slightly salty tomato sauce is a savory Greek specialty. It pairs beautifully with Dilled Persian Rice (page 233).

1 small onion, chopped	¼ teaspoon salt
¼ cup white wine	1¼ pounds large or medium
2½ cups chopped fresh tomatoes	shrimp in shells, peeled and
(1½ pounds whole)	deveined (or 1 pound peeled
2 tablespoons chopped fresh	and deveined)
parsley	2 ounces feta cheese, crumbled
½ teaspoon dried oregano	2 tablespoons chopped fresh
½ teaspoon crushed red pepper	basil

1. In a 2-quart saucepan cook the onion in the wine until the onion is translucent. Add the tomatoes, parsley, oregano, red pepper, and salt, and cook on low heat for 10 minutes.

2. Add the shrimp, and cook until they turn pink, about 2–3 minutes. Stir in the cheese and let it melt. Sprinkle with fresh basil and serve.

Yield: Serves 4

Each serving has approximately 233 calories, 33 g. protein, 6 g. total fat (2.2 g. unsaturated fat, 2.6 g. saturated fat), 10 g. carbohydrates, 228 mg. cholesterol, 2.4 g. fiber, 513 mg. sodium, 190 mg. calcium. Exchanges per serving: 4 meat, ½ vegetable.

Zuppa di Pesce

A mélange of tender seafood and vegetables in a tomato-fish broth.

½ teaspoon fennel seeds
½ tablespoon olive oil
1 medium onion, finely chopped
3 garlic cloves, finely chopped
1 large green bell pepper, seeded, cored, and chopped
1 small red bell pepper, seeded, cored, and chopped
½ teaspoon saffron
2 pounds fresh plum tomatoes, cored, seeded, and pureed
2 tablespoons Ricard or dry sherry
2 cups Basic Fish Stock (page 100)

½ teaspoon crushed red pepper
1 teaspoon fresh thyme or ¾ teaspoon dried
½ cup lightly chopped fresh basil
1 can (6-ounce) tomato paste
½ pound monkfish, trimmed of membrane
½ pound shrimp, peeled and deveined
½ pound sea scallops
12 clams, washed well in cold water
12 mussels, washed well in cold water

1. Sauté the fennel seeds in a dry, heavy cast-iron pan until they crackle and brown slightly, about 3 minutes. Grind seeds with a mortar and pestle. (The roasting makes grinding easier.)

2. In a 6-quart pot, heat the oil and sauté the onion, garlic, green and red peppers, and saffron for 5 minutes.

3. Add the plum tomato puree, and cook for 10 minutes. Add the sherry, stock, red pepper, thyme, and basil, and cook for 3 minutes. Add the tomato paste and monkfish, and cook for 5 minutes. Add the shrimp, scallops, clams, and mussels, and cook, covered, for 5 more minutes.

Yield: Serves 8

Each serving has approximately 183 calories, 23 g. protein, 6.3 g. total fat (2.5 g. unsaturated fat, 0.7 g. saturated fat), 13.6 g. carbohydrates, 85.6 mg. cholesterol, 3.6 g. fiber, 175 mg. sodium, 86 mg. calcium. Exchanges per serving: ¼ fat, 2⅓ meat, 2 vegetable.

Ceviche with Chunky Vegetable Salsa

A tangy refreshing fish dish that "cooks" in fresh citrus juices, served with a spicy Mexican salsa. It's also good with Green Tomatillo Sauce (page 130).

1 pound sole fillets, sliced very thin
½ cup fresh lime juice
½ cup plus 1 tablespoon fresh lemon juice
5 ounces Italian plum tomatoes to make 1 cup chopped tomatoes (3 or 4 tomatoes)
½ medium zucchini, finely chopped

¼ cup finely chopped ripe avocado
1 small cayenne or jalapeño pepper, finely chopped
1 large garlic clove, finely chopped
1 teaspoon fresh sage, finely chopped
⅛ teaspoon salt
8 leaves romaine lettuce

1. Lay the fish fillets in a shallow glass dish in one layer, pour the lime juice and ½ cup of the lemon juice over them, making sure the juices completely cover the fish. Cover with plastic wrap, and refrigerate for 4 hours. The fish will become white and will look cooked.

2. Meanwhile, core, seed, and chop the tomatoes. Transfer them to a separate bowl, and add the remaining tablespoon of lemon juice, the zucchini, avocado, pepper, garlic, sage, and salt to make the Mexican salsa.

3. To serve the fish, place the lettuce decoratively on individual salad plates or on a large serving platter. With a spatula, lay the fish fillets on the lettuce, discarding the citrus juices. Spoon the salsa over the fish.

Yield: Serves 4

Each serving has approximately 156 calories, 23 g. protein, 3.6 g. total fat (2.2 g. unsaturated fat, 0.7 g. saturated fat), 10 g. carbohydrates, 54 mg. cholesterol, 2.7 g. fiber, 182 mg. sodium, 43 mg. calcium. Exchanges per serving: 3 meat, 1 vegetable.

Fowl

Chicken with Tarragon Sauce
Chicken with Artichokes and
  Peppers
Chicken Paprikash
Chicken Fettuccine with
  Broccoli
Tandoori Chicken
Marinated Chicken with
  Sautéed Leeks
Chicken Stew with Fresh Herbs
Spicy Chicken with Basil and
  Rice Noodles
Chicken Stir-Fry with Hoisin
  Sauce
Chicken Stir-Fry with
  Cantaloupe
Chicken Breasts Stuffed with
  Smoked Mozzarella and
  Basil

Barbecued Chicken Legs
Pecan-Coated Chicken
Poached Chicken in Mango
  Cream Sauce
Chicken Tostada
Chicken Enchiladas
Curried Chicken Crepes
Moo Shoo Chicken
Indonesian Chicken Satay
Spicy Chicken Coconut Kabobs
Turkey with Cranberry
  Orange Sauce
Turkey Moussaka
Thai Turkey with Eggplant
Turkey-Stuffed Peppers

Chicken with Tarragon Sauce

Tender, tart, peppery chicken in a spicy citrus-flavored sauce.

1 tablespoon margarine
¾ cup chopped onion (1 medium)
3 garlic cloves, chopped
2 tablespoons chopped fresh tarragon or 2 teaspoons dried
4 chicken breast halves, skinned and all fat removed (about 2 pounds)
¼ teaspoon salt
½ teaspoon ground black pepper
1 cup plus 2 tablespoons Basic Chicken Stock (page 86)

2 carrots, peeled, sliced in half lengthwise, then cut into 2-inch pieces
¼ cup dry white wine
3 tablespoons lime or lemon juice
1 tablespoon Worcestershire sauce
1 teaspoon Dijon mustard
1 tablespoon cornstarch

1. In a heavy 4-quart saucepan melt the margarine. Add the onion, garlic, and tarragon, and cook for 1 minute.

2. Sprinkle the chicken breasts with salt and pepper, add them to the pan, and cook for 3 minutes. Transfer the chicken temporarily to a plate while you deglaze the pan by adding ¼ cup of stock to the pan, and scraping the bottom to incorporate the flavorful drippings. Return the chicken breast halves to the pan on their uncooked sides, and cook for 3 more minutes. Again remove the chicken to a plate.

3. Stir in ¾ cup of the stock, the carrots, wine, citrus juice, Worcestershire sauce, and mustard.

4. In a small bowl mix the cornstarch with the remaining 2 tablespoons of chicken stock, and stir it into the sauce.

5. Return the chicken to the saucepan, and cook for 5 minutes, covered, over very low heat.

Yield: Serves 4

Each serving has approximately 218 calories, 25.7 g. protein, 6.7 g. total fat (4.2 g. unsaturated fat, 1.5 g. saturated fat), 11 g. carbohydrates, 79.6 mg. cholesterol, 2 g. fiber, 327 mg. sodium, 64 mg. calcium.

Exchanges per serving: 3½ meat, 1 vegetable.

Chicken with Artichokes and Peppers

Sweet peppers, slightly salty artichoke hearts, and tender chicken in an easy-to-make casserole you can preassemble, refrigerate, and bake at your convenience.

1 tablespoon corn oil	2 garlic cloves, finely chopped
1 tablespoon chopped fresh thyme or teaspoon dried	1 medium red bell pepper, cored, seeded, and cut into strips
4 4-ounce boneless, skinless chicken breasts, fat removed	1 can (15-ounce) artichoke hearts in brine, drained
½ teaspoon freshly ground pepper	2 tablespoons dry white wine
½ cup finely chopped onion (1 small onion)	¼ teaspoon salt

1. Preheat oven to 375° F.

2. In a non-stick 8-inch skillet heat the oil, then add the thyme and chicken breasts. Sprinkle ¼ teaspoon of the pepper over the chicken and cook for 1 minute over medium heat, then turn the chicken over, sprinkle with the remaining ¼ teaspoon pepper, and cook for another minute. Remove the chicken from the pan and set aside, retaining the cooking juices in the pan.

3. Add the onion and garlic to the pan, and sauté for 1 minute. Add the sweet bell pepper, artichokes, wine, and salt, and cook for 1 more minute.

4. Spoon half the vegetables into an 8-inch casserole, place the chicken breasts over them in one layer, and cover them with the rest of the vegetables. Bake for 18–20 minutes.

To microwave, cook the casserole on high, covered, for 9 minutes, rotating the casserole after 4½ minutes.

Yield: Serves 4

Each serving has approximately 224 calories, 30 g. protein, 5.5 g. total fat (3.8 g. unsaturated fat, 1 g. saturated fat), 13.6 g. carbohydrates, 65.3 mg. cholesterol, 9 g. fiber, 264 mg. sodium, 54 mg. calcium. Exchanges per serving: 3½ meat, 1½ vegetable.

Chicken Paprikash

Creamy and sweet, a low-calorie rendition of a favorite Hungarian dish.

1 tablespoon sherry	¼ teaspoon freshly ground
⅓ cup unsalted fat-free chicken	black pepper
stock	4 4-ounce boneless, skinless
1 medium onion, sliced	chicken breasts, fat removed
2 medium garlic cloves, finely	¾ cup plain non-fat yogurt
chopped	¼ cup reduced-fat sour cream
¼ pound fresh mushrooms,	1½ tablespoons sweet Hungarian
sliced	paprika
¼ teaspoon salt	

1. In a small bowl combine the sherry and chicken stock.
2. In a 10-inch non-stick fry pan, brown the onions, garlic, and mushrooms by adding 1 tablespoon of the combined liquid, stirring until the pan dries, then repeating with another tablespoon of liquid. The pan will be slightly dry. Season the vegetables with salt and pepper. Transfer the vegetables to a plate and set the pan aside.
3. Pound the chicken breasts to ¼-inch thickness.
4. In a small bowl combine the yogurt, sour cream, and paprika.
5. Reheat the 10-inch pan, adding 2 tablespoons of the combined liquid. Lay the chicken pieces in the pan and cook on medium-high heat for 2 minutes. Turn the chicken over, add the remaining 2 table-spoons of the liquid to the pan, and cook the chicken for a final 2 or 3 minutes. Reduce heat to low.
6. Stir 1 tablespoon of the hot stock from the pan into the yogurt mixture, then pour the yogurt over the chicken pieces, stirring to coat them well. Heat for 1 minute. Stir in the onions and mushrooms, and cook for 1 more minute.

Yield: Serves 4

Each serving has approximately 223 calories, 29 g. protein, 6.5 g. total fat (2.2 g. unsaturated fat, 1 g. saturated fat), 10 g. carbohydrates, 80 mg. cholesterol, 1.6 g. fiber, 271 mg. sodium, 116 mg. calcium. Exchanges per serving: 3½ meat, ¼ milk, ½ vegetable.

Chicken Fettuccine with Broccoli

Strips of tender chicken and firm broccoli florets in a smooth and creamy cheese sauce. Add a salad, and you have a meal.

1½	pound boneless, skinless chicken breasts, cut into 1½ × ½-inch strips	1	teaspoon margarine
2	shallots or 2 tablespoons onion, finely chopped	2	teaspoons unbleached white flour
1	tablespoon dry white wine	10	ounces skim milk
½	teaspoon ground white pepper	1½	ounces grated Parmesan cheese
3	ounces uncooked fettuccine noodles	1	tablespoon chopped fresh basil or 1 teaspoon dried
3	cups broccoli florets	⅛	teaspoon salt

1. In a 2-quart saucepan, cook the chicken and shallots or onion in the wine for 3 to 4 minutes, or until the chicken turns from pink to white in the center. Remove pan from heat. Sprinkle pepper over chicken breasts, and transfer them to a plate and set aside.

2. In a 3$quart pot cook the fettuccine for 12 minutes in 2 quarts of boiling water. Drain through a colander and set aside.

3. Steam the broccoli for 3 minutes, or microwave in a microwave-safe dish with 1 tablespoon of water on high for 3 minutes, covered. Drain excess liquid when cooked.

4. In the 2-quart saucepan, melt the margarine, stir in the flour, and let cook for 2 minutes, stirring continuously. Add the milk, a little at a time, whisking well until the mixture is smooth. Stir in the cheese and let it melt. Add the basil and salt.

5. Fold the chicken and broccoli into the cheese sauce, and cook on low heat for 1 minute. Add the noodles, stir carefully to coat the noodles, and cook on low for 1 minute. Serve immediately.

Yield: Makes 4 1½-cup servings

Each serving has approximately 257 calories, 24 g. protein, 7 g. total fat (3.3 g. unsaturated fat, 3 g. saturated fat), 24 g. carbohydrates, 69 mg. cholesterol, 3.8 g. fiber, 376 mg. sodium, 289 mg. calcium. Exchanges per serving: 2½ meat, ¼ milk, 1 starch, 1 vegetable.

Tandoori Chicken

A full day of marinating keeps the chicken moist and spicy. If you're a serious curry lover, serve it with Spinach Sag Paneer (page 216) for an all-Indian meal.

2 garlic cloves, chopped	½ teaspoon cayenne pepper
½ tablespoon ground coriander	1 teaspoon turmeric
1 teaspoon ground cumin	2 tablespoons chopped coriander
8 ounces non-fat yogurt	leaves
1 tablespoon chopped fresh	½ teaspoon salt
ginger	4 4-ounce boneless, skinless
1 tablespoon lime juice	chicken breasts, fat removed

1. In a large bowl combine the garlic, coriander, cumin, yogurt, ginger, lime juice, cayenne pepper, turmeric, coriander leaves, and salt. Add the chicken and marinate for 24 hours. Remove the chicken and discard the marinade.

2. Adjust the cooking rack to its second level from the heat, and preheat the broiler or grill.

3. Lay the chicken on a broiling pan and broil 5 minutes per side.

Yield: Serves 4

Each serving has approximately 177 calories, 28 g. protein, 4 g. total fat (2 g. unsaturated fat, 1 g. saturated fat), 6.4 g. carbohydrates, 80.6 mg. cholesterol, 0.4 g. fiber, 400 mg. sodium, 143 mg. calcium. Exchanges per serving: 3 meat, ¼ milk.

Marinated Chicken with Sautéed Leeks

Sweet taste and smooth texture of leeks top spicily marinated chicken.

Marinade for chicken:

1 8-ounce cup salt-free tomato sauce
2 garlic cloves
1 teaspoon chopped fresh mint
½ teaspoon chopped fresh ginger
¼ teaspoon cinnamon
½ teaspoon sugar
½ teaspoon low-sodium soy sauce
½ teaspoon chili powder

4 4-ounce boneless, skinless chicken breasts, fat removed
1 leek
2 tablespoons water
½ tablespoon margarine
⅛ teaspoon salt

1. Combine all marinade ingredients in food processor or blender and blend until smooth.

2. Pound chicken breasts to ¼-inch thickness, and lay them in a wide flat dish. Pour the marinade over and let the chicken marinate for 2 hours, refrigerated.

3. Place the cooking rack at the second level from the heat, and preheat the broiler or grill.

4. Meanwhile, trim the root and green section from the leek and slice it in half lengthwise. Wash carefully to remove any soil. Cut into ¼-inch slices.

5. In an 8-inch sauté pan cook the leek with 2 tablespoons of water over medium heat for 4 or 5 minutes, or until the leek softens and the water evaporates. Add margarine and salt, and stir until the margarine melts and coats the leek slices. Keep warm.

6. While the leek cooks, broil or grill the chicken for 4½ minutes on each side.

7. To serve, spoon some of the sautéed leeks over each chicken breast.

Yield: Serves 4

Each serving has approximately 185 calories, 25.6 g. protein, 5.2 g. total fat (3.1 g. unsaturated fat, 1.2 g. saturated fat), 9 g. carbohydrates, 80 mg. cholesterol, 1.5 g. fiber, 547 mg. sodium, 41.4 mg. calcium.

Exchanges per serving: 3 meat, 1 vegetable.

Chicken Stew with Fresh Herbs

Four aromatic herbs and three chewy vegetables flavor this tender chicken stew. If you can't get one of the herbs, add fresh chopped parsley, but don't substitute dried herbs.

2½	pound fryer chicken	⅓	pound mushrooms, cut in half
⅔	pound baking potatoes	½	tablespoon fresh sage
1	medium onion, finely chopped	1	teaspoon fresh marjoram leaves
3	garlic cloves, finely chopped	2	tablespoons fresh dill
3	medium carrots, peeled and cut into 1-inch pieces	2	sprigs fresh thyme
2	celery stalks, cut into 1-inch pieces	½	teaspoon salt
		½	teaspoon pepper

1. In a 6-quart saucepan or soup pot, simmer the chicken in 2 quarts of water for 1 hour, uncovered.

2. Meanwhile, in a separate pot, cook potatoes in 1 quart of water for 40 minutes, covered, or until fork-tender. Set aside.

3. Remove the chicken from the pot, let it cool slightly, and remove all skin. Cut the meat from the chicken breasts, cut off the legs and thighs and any other edible pieces, and set them aside. With a defatting cup or spoon, skim fat off the top of the stock. Set the fat-free stock aside; you will have 2–3 cups.

4. In the same pot, sauté the onion and garlic for 2 minutes. Add the carrots, celery, mushrooms, and 1 cup of the chicken stock. Cook together for 10 minutes over low heat.

5. Add the chicken pieces, herbs, and seasonings, and 1 more cup of the remaining stock, and cook together for 10 minutes, uncovered, over low heat.

6. In the meantime, remove the skin from the potatoes. Cut the potatoes into chunks or press them through a ricer. Add the potato chunks directly to the stew and serve, or place ½ cup riced potatoes in individual soup bowls and ladle one-fourth of the chicken and the stock over the riced potatoes.

Yield: Serves 4

Each serving has approximately 258 calories, 28 g. protein, 4 g. total fat (2.1 g. unsaturated fat, 1 g. saturated fat), 27.8 g. carbohydrates, 79.6 mg. cholesterol, 4.6 g. fiber, 399 mg. sodium, 78 mg. calcium.
Exchanges per serving: 3 meat, ½ starch, 2 vegetable.

Spicy Chicken with Basil and Rice Noodles

Chewy chicken and rice noodles lightly coated in a rich basil oyster sauce.

3½ ounces rice noodles
2 garlic cloves, finely chopped
½ tablespoon chopped fresh ginger
½ teaspoon chili flakes
3 teaspoons toasted sesame oil
½ cup lightly chopped fresh basil

2 tablespoons dry sherry (optional)
2 tablespoons oyster sauce
¾ pound cooked boneless, skinless chicken breasts, shredded

1. Put the rice noodles in a bowl, cover with warm water, and soak for 10 minutes. Drain in a colander.

2. In a wok or 10-inch fry pan, sauté the garlic, ginger, and chili flakes with 1 teaspoon of the oil for 1 minute. Add the rice noodles, basil, and sherry, and stir-fry for 1 minute. Add the remaining 2 teaspoons of sesame oil and the oyster sauce, and stir-fry for 1 minute. Add the chicken, and stir-fry for 1 more minute.

Yield: Serves 4

Each serving has approximately 275 calories, 26.7 g. protein, 6.5 g. total fat (4.5 g. unsaturated fat, 1.4 g. saturated fat), 23.7 g. carbohydrates, 72.2 mg. cholesterol, 0.4 g. fiber, 221 mg. sodium, 36.7 mg. calcium.
Exchanges per serving: 3 meat, ½ starch.

Chicken Stir-Fry with Hoisin Sauce

A lightly spiced, slightly sweet dish with strips of chewy chicken and crunchy vegetables.

1 tablespoon cornstarch	1 small red bell pepper, cored, seeded, and cut into thin strips
¼ cup cold water	
2 tablespoons hoisin sauce	1 zucchini, cut into strips ¼ × ¼ × 2 inches
1 tablespoon toasted sesame oil	
3 garlic cloves, finely chopped	3½ ounces oyster mushrooms, trimmed of stems and halved
½ tablespoon finely chopped fresh ginger	3 scallions, cut into diagonal slices 1 inch thick
2 hot Szechuan peppers, finely chopped	
1 pound boneless, skinless chicken breasts, fat removed and cut into 1½ × ½-inch strips	

1. In a small bowl dissolve the cornstarch in water, then stir in the hoisin sauce. Set aside.

2. In a wok or non-stick 10-inch fry pan, heat the oil over medium heat. Add the garlic, ginger, and Szechuan peppers, and cook together for 30 seconds.

3. Add the chicken, and cook for 2–3 minutes, stirring frequently, until the chicken turns from pink to white. Move the chicken strips to the sides of the pan, creating a well in the center.

4. Add the bell pepper and zucchini strips to the center of the pan, and cook for 1 minute, stirring frequently. Move them to the side of the pan.

5. Add the mushrooms, then the scallions to the well, cook for 1 minute, then move them aside.

6. Stir the cornstarch mixture, pour it in the well, and cook, stirring until it thickens. Stir the chicken and vegetables into the sauce until they are well coated.

Yield: Serves 4

Each serving has approximately 205 calories, 27.7 g. protein, 5.4 g. total fat (3.8 g. unsaturated fat, 1 g. saturated fat), 11.2 g. carbohydrates, 65.3 mg. cholesterol, 1.8 g. fiber, 227 mg. sodium, 27 mg. calcium.

Exchanges per serving: 3 meat, ⅛ starch, 1 vegetable.

Chicken Stir-Fry with Cantaloupe

Many tastes and textures in this oriental dish — chewy chicken, sweet and juicy cantaloupe, crunchy peas and scallions, plus a hint of hot peppers and tangy ginger.

2 teaspoons low-sodium soy sauce
2 teaspoons oyster sauce
2 tablespoons cold, fat-free chicken stock
1 tablespoon cornstarch
2 tablespoons cold water
2 teaspoons lime juice
1 tablespoon safflower oil
2 teaspoons fresh ginger, finely chopped
2 garlic cloves, finely chopped

¼ teaspoon crushed red pepper flakes
1 pound boneless, skinless chicken breasts, cut into 1½ × ½-inch strips
3 ounces snow peas, stems removed then cut diagonally into ½-inch slices
1½ cups fresh cantaloupe pieces, about ½ × 1 inch
4 scallions, cut diagonally into 1-inch pieces

1. In a small bowl, combine the soy sauce, oyster sauce, chicken stock, cornstarch, cold water, and lime juice. Mix well until the cornstarch dissolves. Set aside.

2. In a wok or 10-inch fry pan, heat the oil over medium heat, add the ginger, garlic, and red pepper flakes, and cook together for 30 seconds. Add the chicken pieces and, stirring frequently, cook for 2–3 minutes, or until the chicken turns from pink to white. Move the chicken to the side of the wok or pan, add the snow peas, and cook for 1 minute, then add the cantaloupe pieces and scallions, and cook for 1 more minute.

3. Move all the cooked food to the sides of the pan, creating a well in which to cook the sauce. Stir the cornstarch mixture, then pour it in the center of the pan and cook, stirring frequently, until the cornstarch thickens. Pull the chicken and vegetables into the well and coat them with the cornstarch mixture.

Yield: Serves 4

Each serving has approximately 200 calories, 27.7 g. protein, 5.1 g. total fat (3.7 g. unsaturated fat, 0.7 g. saturated fat), 10.1 g. carbohydrates, 65.3 mg. cholesterol, 1.4 g. fiber, 231 mg. sodium, 38 mg. calcium.

Exchanges per serving: ¼ fruit, 3 meat, ½ vegetable.

Chicken Breasts Stuffed with Smoked Mozzarella and Basil

Creamy smoked cheese and fresh basil encased in tender chicken with a crisp and grainy crust.

4 4-ounce boneless, skinless chicken breasts, thinly sliced	½ teaspoon freshly ground black pepper
½ cup plain bread crumbs	2½ ounces smoked mozzarella, coarsely chopped
1½ tablespoons chopped fresh thyme or ¾ teaspoon dried	1 small bunch fresh basil (about 30 leaves)
½ teaspoon paprika	

1. Preheat oven to 375° F.
2. Wash the chicken breasts and pat dry. Pound them lightly with a wooden mallet until each one is ¼ inch thick.
3. Combine the bread crumbs, thyme, paprika, and pepper in a cup, and pour onto a piece of foil.
4. One by one, dip each piece of chicken into the bread crumb mixture, coating both sides. You'll only use about half the bread crumbs, but it's easier to work with an ample supply.
5. Put one-fourth of the smoked mozzarella and the basil leaves in the center of each piece of chicken, then roll them up, and lay them in a bake-and-serve dish, seam side down. Bake for 20 minutes, uncovered.

Yield: Serves 4

Each serving has approximately 210 calories, 31 g. protein, 6.3 g. total fat (2.3 g. unsaturated fat, 3.2 g. saturated fat), 5.8 g. carbohydrates, 81 mg. cholesterol, 0.9 g. fiber, 205 mg. sodium, 143 mg. calcium. Exchanges per serving: 3½ meat, ¼ starch.

Barbecued Chicken Legs

Tender, chewy, spicy, and sweet.

12 chicken legs (about 3 pounds)	1 cup (½ recipe) Barbecue Sauce (page 128)
3 tablespoons unbleached flour	

1. Preheat oven to 375° F.

2. Remove the chicken skin by peeling the skin toward the bony end of the leg, then, using a dry paper towel, pull the skin over the bone and off the leg.

3. Dredge each chicken leg lightly in flour, shaking off excess. Place on a baking pan, and bake for 10 minutes.

4. Brush the legs with ½ cup of the barbecue sauce, and bake for 10 more minutes.

5. Brush the legs with ¼ cup of the sauce, and bake for 10 more minutes. Remove the pan from the oven and preheat the broiler. Brush the chicken with the remaining ¼ cup of the sauce, and broil the legs for 3 minutes on the mid-shelf of the broiler.

Yield: Serves 4

Each serving has approximately 237 calories, 31.5 g. protein, 6.5 g. total fat (4 g. unsaturated fat, 1.6 g. saturated fat), 11.5 g. carbohydrates, 99 mg. cholesterol, 1 g. fiber, 196 mg. sodium, 32 mg. calcium. Exchanges per serving: 3½ meat, ⅙ starch, 1 vegetable.

Pecan-Coated Chicken

Crisp, nutty crust encasing tender chicken in an easy-to-make dish.

3½ tablespoons pecans	4 4-ounce boneless, skinless chicken breasts, trimmed of fat
2 tablespoons bread crumbs	1 teaspoon corn oil

1. Preheat the broiler, and set the broiler rack at the second level from the source of heat.

2. In a food processor or blender grind the pecans and bread crumbs together until fine. Lay a piece of foil or wax paper on the counter top, and transfer the breading mixture to it.

3. Dip each chicken piece into the breading, coating both sides.

4. Lightly coat a non-stick 10-inch skillet with 1 teaspoon of oil, and preheat it over medium heat. Add the chicken pieces and pan-fry on each side for 1 minute.

5. Transfer the breaded chicken pieces to a broiler pan, and broil for 2 minutes, turn the chicken over, and broil for 2 more minutes.

Yield: Serves 4

Each serving has approximately 190 calories, 27 g. protein, 7.1 g. total fat (5.5 g. unsaturated fat, 1 g. saturated fat), 3.5 g. carbohydrates, 65.5 mg. cholesterol, 0.6 g. fiber, 96 mg. sodium, 19 mg. calcium. Exchanges per serving: ¼ fat, 3 meat, ⅕ starch.

Poached Chicken in Mango Cream Sauce

Strips of tender chicken at room-temperature and a slightly tart and fruity sauce in a beautifully arranged summer dish.

2½ cups Basic Chicken Stock (page 86)	1 cup Mango Cream Sauce (page 139)
½ teaspoon salt	1½ tablespoons plain non-fat yogurt
4 4-ounce boneless, skinless breasts of chicken, trimmed of fat	12 basil or cilantro (coriander) leaves, or a small bunch of watercress for garnish

1. In a 10-inch sauté pan, heat the stock and salt to a low simmer, then turn heat as low as possible, add the chicken, and cook without rippling the stock for 4 minutes on each side.

2. Cut each chicken breast across the grain (across the width) into 6 short strips. If still pink in the center, return the strips to the poaching liquid until they lose their color. Lay the chicken strips on paper towels to remove excess moisture.

3. Spread ¼ cup of the mango cream sauce in a circle in the center of each of 4 small individual plates. On each plate lay 6 strips of chicken over the sauce in a spoke pattern emanating from the center.

4. In a small bowl, mix the yogurt with a fork until creamy and smooth. Dip a toothpick in the yogurt, and between every piece of chicken make a quick long stroke about ¾ inch long in the mango cream sauce to add yogurt "spokes" to the design. Place a garnish of basil leaves, cilantro, or watercress in the center of each plate.

Yield: Serves 4

Each serving has approximately 166 calories, 27 g. protein, 1.6 g. total fat (0.7 g. unsaturated fat, 0.4 g. saturated fat), 10.4 g. carbohydrates, 65.6 mg. cholesterol, 2 g. fiber, 349 mg. sodium, 45 mg. calcium. Exchanges per serving: ½ fruit, 3 meat.

Chicken Tostada

Crunchy, spicy, meaty, and chewy—lots of tastes and textures on a crisp tortilla.

4   corn tortillas
8   ounces cooked chicken meat, shredded (about 1½ cups)
⅔   cup Spicy Salsa (page 129)
¼   cup grated part-skim mozzarella cheese (1 ounce)

4   tablespoons scallions, finely sliced
¼   cup plain non-fat yogurt

1. Preheat oven to 450° F.
2. Lay the tortillas on a baking pan and toast for 10 minutes. Set aside.
3. Mix the chicken meat with the salsa, and spread it over the toasted tortillas. Sprinkle the grated cheese on each tortilla, then the scallions, and finally, put a tablespoon of yogurt on each. Serve immediately.

Yield: Serves 4

Each serving has approximately 197 calories, 21.7 g. protein, 5 g. total fat (3 g. unsaturated fat, 1.3 g. saturated fat), 16.3 g. carbohydrates, 50 mg. cholesterol, 3 g. fiber, 109 mg. sodium, 109 mg. calcium. Exchanges per serving: 2 meat, 1 starch, ½ vegetable.

Chicken Enchiladas

Chewy chicken shreds and spicy sauce wrapped in a soft corn tortilla and drizzled with cheese.

10 ounces cooked chicken, shredded (about 2 cups)
4   scallions, finely chopped

2½ cups Enchilada Sauce (page 130)
8   6-inch prepared corn tortillas
1½ ounces part-skim mozzarella cheese, grated

1. Preheat oven to 400° F., unless you have a microwave.
2. In a bowl, combine the chicken, half the scallions, and ½ cup of the enchilada sauce.

3. Soften the corn tortillas, two at a time, by steaming them for 10 seconds, or cook in a microwave for 10 seconds on high.

4. Spoon 1 cup of the enchilada sauce on the bottom of a 9 × 11-inch pan. Fill each tortilla with about ¼ cup of the chicken mixture. Roll each tortilla and place seam side down on the sauce in the pan. Top with the remaining cup of enchilada sauce, sprinkle with the cheese and the remaining scallions. Bake for 10 minutes or microwave on high for 5 minutes.

Yield: Serves 8

Each serving has approximately 151 calories, 15 g. protein, 3.4 g. total fat (2 g. unsaturated fat, 1 g. saturated fat), 16 g. carbohydrates, 33 mg. cholesterol, 3.3 g. fiber, 65 mg. sodium, 95 mg. calcium.
Exchanges per serving: 1½ meat, ⅔ starch, ½ vegetable.

Curried Chicken Crepes

A creamy curry sauce napping curried chicken, sweet raisins, and mushrooms.

1 recipe Perfect Crepes (page 265)	*Curry Sauce:*
1¼ pounds skinless, boneless chicken breasts, fat removed	1½ tablespoons chopped shallots
2 cups Basic Chicken Stock (page 86)	2 tablespoons dry white wine
3½ ounces shiitake mushrooms, trimmed of lower stems	1 tablespoon margarine
¼ cup golden raisins	1 tablespoon flour
¼ teaspoon freshly ground black pepper	10 ounces skim milk
⅔ cup lightly chopped watercress	⅛ teaspoon salt
	¼ teaspoon freshly ground black pepper
	¾ teaspoon curry powder
	8 sprigs watercress, for garnish

1. Preheat oven to 350° F., and lightly coat an 8 × 14-inch bake-and-serve pan with non-stick cooking spray.

2. Make crepes and set them aside.

3. Pound the chicken lightly with a wooden mallet to ¼-inch thickness.

4. In a 10-inch non-stick fry pan heat the chicken stock to a low

simmer. Add the chicken, reduce the heat until there is no movement in the stock, and cook for 3 minutes. The chicken should be barely pink in the center. Remove the chicken and set aside to cool for about 5 minutes. Discard the stock or save it for soup.

5. Using the same fry pan, sauté the mushrooms and raisins for 2 minutes.

6. Cut the chicken into thin strips about 2½ inches by ¼ inch, and add them to the pan, along with the pepper and watercress, and continue cooking for 2 more minutes. Transfer the chicken-mushroom mixture to a bowl and set aside while you make the curry sauce.

7. Rinse the fry pan and return it to the burner. Add the shallots and wine, and cook for 2 minutes over medium heat. Add the margarine, and when it has melted, sprinkle in the flour and stir to incorporate it. Reduce the heat to low and cook for 1 minute. Add the milk slowly, 2 tablespoons at a time, stirring as the sauce thickens. Season with the salt, pepper, and curry powder, and cook for 1 more minute. Remove from heat.

8. Mix ¼ cup of the curry sauce into the chicken-mushroom mixture, and stir to coat.

9. Place ⅓ cup of the chicken-mushroom mixture down the center of a crepe. Turn one side of the crepe over the filling and continue rolling the crepe up. Repeat the procedure for the remaining crepes.

10. Lay the crepes seam side down in the prepared baking pan, cover with foil, and bake for 15 minutes. Remove the foil, drizzle the remaining sauce over the crepes, and bake for 5 more minutes. Garnish the serving dish with sprigs of watercress.

Yield: Serves 8

Each serving has approximately 195 calories, 20.5 g. protein, 4 g. total fat (1.7 g. unsaturated fat, 0.9 g. saturated fat), 18.3 g. carbohydrates, 41.4 mg. cholesterol, 1.7 g. fiber, 213 mg. sodium, 65.9 mg. calcium. Exchanges per serving: ¼ fat, ¼ fruit, 1½ meat, 1 starch.

Moo Shoo Chicken

This is an oriental dish full of many textures — crunchy bamboo shoots, tender chewy chicken, and wispy lily flowers in a sweet hoisin sauce. Serve it over rice or roll 2–3 tablespoons up in packaged Chinese pancakes with a little hoisin sauce. You'll find the oriental ingredients in oriental markets.

2 cups cooked chicken, skin removed, shredded	1 can (8 ounces) bamboo shoots, drained
1 tablespoon low-sodium soy sauce	3 egg whites
1 tablespoon dry sherry (optional)	1 tablespoon toasted sesame oil
1 teaspoon cornstarch	2 garlic cloves, finely chopped
1 tablespoon water	2 slices fresh ginger, finely chopped
30 dried Chinese lily flowers	¼ cup unsalted, fat-free chicken stock
2 tablespoons dried wood ear mushrooms	1 tablespoon hoisin sauce
	3 scallions, finely chopped

1. Combine the cooked chicken, soy sauce, sherry, cornstarch, and water in a bowl. Let marinate for ½ hour.

2. Meanwhile, soak the lily flowers and wood ear mushrooms in 2 cups of warm water in a bowl for 20 minutes. Cut the bamboo shoots into thin strips, and set aside.

3. In a non-stick fry pan cook the egg whites over medium heat for 1 minute, or until coagulated. Shred and set aside.

4. Shred the lily flowers by pulling from top to bottom with your fingers. Set aside.

5. Heat the oil in a wok or large fry pan. Add the garlic and ginger, and cook for 1 minute over medium-high heat. Add the chicken, bamboo shoots, lily flowers, and mushrooms, and cook together for 2 minutes. Add the stock, cooked egg whites, hoisin sauce, and the scallions. Stir together and cook for 2 more minutes.

Yield: Serves 8

Each serving has approximately 141 calories, 20 g. protein, 3.9 g. total fat (2.6 g. unsaturated fat, 0.8 g. saturated fat), 5.6 g. carbohydrates, 48 mg. cholesterol, 1.2 g. fiber, 176 mg. sodium, 11 mg. calcium. Exchanges per serving: 3 meat, ½ vegetable.

Indonesian Chicken Satay

Nutty, mildly spicy, with the piquant flavor of the Far East, this delightful dish is excellent with rice or bulgur. If you want to serve it as an appetizer, divide the recipe among twice as many skewers.

Marinade:

½ small onion, finely chopped
1 garlic clove, finely chopped
½ tablespoon fresh chopped ginger
¾ cup Basic Chicken Stock (page 86)
2 tablespoons lime juice
1 teaspoon Tabasco
¾ teaspoon red pepper flakes
⅓ cup peanut butter
2 teaspoons brown sugar
1 teaspoon low-sodium soy sauce

1 pound boneless, skinless chicken breasts, fat removed
8 skewers

1. In a blender or food processor combine the marinade ingredients and puree until smooth.

2. Cut the chicken into 1-inch pieces. Place them in a 1-quart bowl, then pour the marinade over the chicken, stirring to coat each piece. Marinate the chicken for at least 2 hours. If you are using bamboo skewers, soak them in water for half an hour.

3. Preheat broiler.

4. Divide and thread the chicken pieces on the skewers. Discard the marinade. Place the skewers on a broiling pan on the second rack from the source of heat, and broil or grill for 2½ minutes, then turn the skewers over and broil for another 2½ minutes.

Yield: Serves 4

Each serving has approximately 171 calories, 28.3 g. protein, 5 g. total fat (3.5 g. unsaturated fat, 1 g. saturated fat), 2.6 g. carbohydrates, 65 mg. cholesterol, 0.5 g. fiber, 180 mg. sodium, 18 mg. calcium. Exchanges per serving: 3½ meat.

Spicy Chicken Coconut Kabobs

Bites of tender chicken marinated in hot Thai seasoning that you buy in oriental grocery stores in small cans.

2 tablespoons grated lime peel	2 scallions, finely chopped
4 garlic cloves, finely chopped	1½ pounds boneless, skinless
2 teaspoons Thai chili paste	chicken breasts, cut into
1 cup plain non-fat yogurt	1-inch squares
½ teaspoon coconut extract	2 tablespoons grated coconut
4 teaspoons apple juice	(garnish)
concentrate	

1. Put the grated lime peel, garlic, chili paste, yogurt, coconut extract, apple juice, and scallions in blender or food processor, and blend to make a smooth marinade.

2. Pour the marinade over the chicken pieces and marinate for 2 hours.

3. Preheat broiler, and place broiling rack on second level from the source of heat.

4. Divide the chicken pieces among eight 8-inch skewers, about 4 pieces per skewer. Lay the skewers on a broiling pan, sprinkle half the coconut on top, and broil for 5 minutes. Turn and baste the other side with the marinade, sprinkle with remaining coconut, then broil for 5 more minutes.

Yield: Makes 4 two-skewer servings

Each serving has approximately 248 calories, 42.6 g. protein, 3.8 g. total fat (1.1 g. unsaturated fat, 2 g. saturated fat), 9 g. carbohydrates, 99 mg. cholesterol, 0.9 g. fiber, 153 mg. sodium, 150 mg. calcium. Exchanges per serving: ¼ fat, 4 meat, ⅓ milk.

Turkey with Cranberry Orange Sauce

Sautéed turkey slices smothered in tart, sweet cranberries.

1 pound boneless, skinless turkey breasts
1½ cups fresh uncooked cranberries
⅓ cup orange juice concentrate
⅓ cup water
1 teaspoon grated orange peel

½ tablespoon corn or canola oil
½ cup plus 2 tablespoons unsalted fat-free chicken stock
4 orange slices, each cut in half, for garnish

1. Pound the turkey pieces until they are ½ inch thick. If they are too thick to pound out, slice them in half horizontally first.

2. In a 10-inch non-stick fry pan combine the cranberries, orange juice, water, and orange peel, and cook over medium heat until all the cranberries pop, about 5 minutes. Remove the cranberry mixture to a dish and set aside.

3. In the same pan, heat the oil over medium-high heat for 1 minute. Reduce the heat to medium-low, add the turkey slices, and cook for 2 minutes on each side. Transfer the turkey to a warmed serving plate.

4. With heat on medium-low, add the chicken stock, stirring to deglaze the pan, and cook for 1½ minutes. Add the cranberry mixture to the stock, and heat together for 1 minute. Pour the cranberry mixture over the turkey slices, and garnish with orange slices.

Yield: Serves 4

Each serving has approximately 194 calories, 26.8 g. protein, 3.2 g. total fat (2.2 g. unsaturated fat, 0.5 g. saturated fat), 13.4 g. carbohydrates, 65.3 mg. cholesterol, 1.8 g. fiber, 74 mg. sodium, 22.6 mg. calcium.

Exchanges per serving: ½ fruit, 3 meat.

Turkey Moussaka

Here's how to enjoy all the rich, piquant flavors of a traditional moussaka without all the traditional calories.

2½ medium eggplants	⅓ cup bulgur wheat
2½ teaspoons onion powder	2 egg whites
2½ teaspoons paprika	
1½ medium onions, finely chopped	*White sauce::*
1⅓ pounds lean ground turkey	4 teaspoons corn oil
3 bay leaves	2 tablespoons all-purpose or unbleached flour
2½ tablespoons tomato paste	1⅓ cups skim milk
½ teaspoon ground white pepper	⅛ teaspoon salt
⅛ teaspoon ground nutmeg	⅛ teaspoon nutmeg
2½ teaspoons fresh thyme or 1½ teaspoons dried	⅛ teaspoon white pepper
8 ounces vegetable cocktail or tomato juice	2½ tablespoons grated fresh Parmesan cheese

1. Preheat oven to 375° F.

2. Peel and cut the eggplants crosswise in ¾-inch-thick slices. Sprinkle each side with onion powder and paprika. Line a large baking sheet with foil or parchment paper. Place the eggplant on the baking sheet and bake for 30 minutes. Set the eggplant aside and reduce the oven heat to 325° F.

3. Heat a 12-inch skillet over medium heat. Add the onion and ground turkey, and cook until the onions are soft, about 5 minutes. Add the bay leaves, tomato paste, pepper, nutmeg, and thyme. Sauté, stirring frequently, until the meat is cooked, about 5 minutes. Remove from the heat and discard the bay leaves.

4. In a small pot heat the vegetable or tomato juice to a simmer. Remove from the heat, stir in the bulgur wheat, and let sit for 15 minutes.

5. In another bowl, beat the egg whites until stiff.

6. Add the bulgur-juice mixture and egg whites to the meat, and set aside.

7. To make the white sauce, in an 8-inch skillet heat the oil over low heat. Sprinkle the flour into the oil, stirring to incorporate. Slowly add the milk and, using a wooden spoon or a whisk, stir continually until

the sauce thickens and has no lumps. Season with salt, nutmeg, pepper, and Parmesan cheese. Cook for 1 more minute, and remove from heat.

8. To assemble the dish, layer half the eggplant slices on the bottom of a bake-and-serve dish about 10 × 12 inches. Top with the meat mixture, then cover with the remaining eggplant slices. Pour the sauce on top and bake, uncovered, for 30 minutes.

Yield: Serves 8

Each serving has approximately 253 calories, 20 g. protein, 10.2 g. total fat (6.9 g. unsaturated fat, 3.1 g. saturated fat), 22.3 g. carbohydrates, 46.5 mg. cholesterol, 7 g. fiber, 270 mg. sodium, 159 mg. calcium.

Exchanges per serving: 3 meat, ⅓ starch, 2½ vegetable.

Thai Turkey with Eggplant

Hot and spicy ground meat with chewy tender eggplant.

¼ cup finely chopped onion (about ½ small onion)	1 pound lean ground turkey or chicken
2 garlic cloves, finely chopped	1 tablespoon low-sodium soy sauce
1½ teaspoons finely chopped fresh ginger	1 tablespoon Worcestershire sauce
¼ teaspoon red pepper flakes	½ cup coarsely chopped basil leaves
1 tablespoon dry sherry	
2 tablespoons tomato paste	2 scallions, cut into ¼-inch slices
6 tablespoons water	
1 small round eggplant, about ¾ pound, peeled and cut into ¾-inch cubes	3 tablespoons lime juice

1. In a 10-inch, heavy-gauge fry pan cook the onion, garlic, ginger, and red pepper flakes in the sherry for about 2–3 minutes.

2. Mix the tomato paste with the water, and stir into the pan.

3. Stir in the cubed eggplant and cook on low heat for 3–4 minutes.

4. Add the ground turkey or chicken and continue cooking for 5–6 minutes, stirring frequently. Add the soy sauce, Worcestershire sauce, basil leaves, scallions, and lime juice, and cook for 3–4 more minutes. Serve with rice.

Yield: Serves 4

Each serving has approximately 186 calories, 26.2 g. protein, 3.8 g. total fat (2 g. unsaturated fat, 1 g. saturated fat), 10.8 g. carbohydrates, 80 mg. cholesterol, 3.6 g. fiber, 289 mg. sodium, 65 mg. calcium. Exchanges per serving: 3 meat, 1 vegetable.

Turkey-Stuffed Peppers

Bell pepper boats filled with chewy brown rice, crisp corn kernels, and well-flavored ground turkey.

2 large green or red bell peppers	¾ cup cooked brown rice
½ cup chopped onion (1 small onion)	2 tablespoons Worcestershire sauce
2 garlic cloves, chopped	¼ cup fresh chopped parsley
½ pound lean ground turkey	⅓ teaspoon freshly ground black pepper
2 tablespoons tomato paste	
¾ cup fresh or frozen corn, defrosted	¼ cup grated low-fat mozzarella cheese (1 ounce)

1. Cut the peppers in half lengthwise to form four oval boats, and remove all seeds. Boil them for 5 minutes in 2 quarts of water, or microwave in a microwave-safe bowl, covered with plastic wrap, on high for 5 minutes. Drain and rinse with cold water.

2. In a 10-inch non-stick fry pan, sauté the onion and garlic for 2 minutes. Add the ground turkey, tomato paste, and corn, stirring frequently. Cook for 5 minutes on medium heat. Add the rice, Worcestershire sauce, parsley, and black pepper, and cook for 2 minutes on low heat, stirring occasionally.

3. Fill each pepper boat with one-fourth of the cooked turkey mixture. Sprinkle each pepper with 1 tablespoon of the cheese, and broil or microwave on high for 2 minutes.

Yield: Serves 4

Each serving has approximately 189 calories, 13 g. protein, 6.2 g. total fat (3.6 g. unsaturated fat, 2.3 g. saturated fat), 21.4 g. carbohydrates, 31 mg. cholesterol, 3 g. fiber, 164 mg. sodium, 79 mg. calcium. Exchanges per serving: 2 meat, ⅔ starch, 1 vegetable.

Meat

Brisket of Beef

Eye Round Roast with
Vegetables

Stir-Fry Beef and Broccoli in
Oyster Sauce

Beef with Five-Spice Sauce
and Watercress

21 Alarm Chili

Huevos Rancheros

Veal with Peaches, Brandy,
and Chervil

Veal Loaf

Veal Parmesan

Veal Marsala

Marinated Lamb Kabobs

Lamb and Eggplant Stew

Lamb Stew

Pork Tenderloin with Fennel
and Chestnuts

Pork Tenderloin with
Chutney Glaze

Broiled Ham with Orange
Honey Glaze

Brisket of Beef

Chewy beef, tender vegetables in a richly seasoned sauce.

1	onion, peeled and thinly sliced	½	pound carrots, peeled and cut into 1-inch slices
3	garlic cloves, finely chopped		
2	teaspoons chopped fresh parsley or dill	¼	pound mushrooms, sliced in half
¼	cup red wine	3	bay leaves
1	can (8-ounce) tomato sauce	2	teaspoons fresh thyme or ½ teaspoon dried
1	cup water		
2	teaspoons garlic powder	2	tablespoons chopped fresh basil or ¾ teaspoon dried
2	teaspoons onion powder		
2	teaspoons unbleached flour	¾	teaspoon salt
1	teaspoon paprika	½	teaspoon coarsely ground black pepper
2	pounds brisket, trimmed of all visible fat (1¾ pounds trimmed weight)		

1. Preheat oven to 250° F.

2. In a 10-inch fry pan, cook the onion, garlic, and fresh parsley or dill in 2 tablespoons of the wine for 2 minutes at medium heat. Add the tomato sauce, water, and the remaining 2 tablespoons of wine. Cook over very low heat for 10 minutes, and set aside.

3. In a small bowl combine the garlic powder, onion powder, flour, and paprika. Coat the brisket with this mixture.

4. In a large heavy cast-iron or non-stick fry pan sear the meat for 5 minutes on each side over medium-high heat.

5. Transfer the meat to a carving board, and slice it against the grain ⅛ inch thick. In an 8-inch bake-and-serve dish stand the slices on edge lengthwise, then gently arrange them so that each slice partially covers the next slice, domino fashion. Ladle the cooked sauce around the meat, and add the carrots, mushrooms, bay leaves, thyme, basil, salt, and pepper. Cover and bake for 1½ hours. Remove bay leaves before serving.

Yield: Serves 8

Each serving has approximately 248 calories, 35 g. protein, 8 g. total fat (3.6 g. unsaturated fat, 3 g. saturated fat), 8.8 g. carbohydrates, 79 mg. cholesterol, 2 g. fiber, 453 mg. sodium, 33 mg. calcium. Exchanges per serving: 3½ meat, 2 vegetable.

Eye Round Roast with Vegetables

Chewy beef and chunky vegetables in a rich wine gravy.

2 pounds eye round roast, trimmed of all visible fat

3 medium carrots, peeled and cut into 2-inch pieces

½ pound small new potatoes, cut into eighths

1 medium onion, cut into large chunks

2 celery stalks, cut into 4-inch pieces and halved lengthwise

½ teaspoon freshly ground black pepper

1 tablespoon low-sodium soy sauce

½ cup dry red wine

½ cup beef stock

1 tablespoon cornstarch

¼ cup cold water

½ cup chopped parsley

1. Preheat oven to 325° F.

2. Place the trimmed eye roast in a plastic oven roasting bag. Add all the vegetables, black pepper, soy sauce, wine, and stock. Tie the bag with its plastic piece, and place on a baking pan. Poke a few holes in the top of the bag, and roast for 1 hour.

3. Remove the pan from the oven and let cool for 10–15 minutes. Open the bag while it is in the pan, and transfer the roast to a carving board, and let it rest for 10 minutes.

4. Meanwhile, empty the contents of the bag into the pan, and remove vegetables with a slotted spoon to a plate. Skim the fat from the remaining drippings, spoon some of the drippings over the meat to keep it moist, then heat the rest in a small saucepan.

5. Combine the cornstarch and cold water until smooth. Add to the hot drippings and stir as the gravy thickens.

6. Cut the meat into thin slices against the grain, and lay them on a warmed platter. Arrange the vegetables around the meat, and garnish with chopped parsley. Serve the gravy in a small pitcher or gravy boat.

Yield: Serves 8

Each serving has approximately 185 calories, 20.3 g. protein, 5.5 g. total fat (2.6 g. unsaturated fat, 2 g. saturated fat), 10.3 g. carbohydrates, 55.4 mg. cholesterol, 1.4 g. fiber, 189 mg. sodium, 19 mg. calcium.

Exchanges per serving: 3 meat, 1 vegetable.

Stir-Fry Beef and Broccoli in Oyster Sauce

Crunchy broccoli florets and chewy beef strips in a rich oriental sauce that's not sweet or spicy.

1 pound sirloin steak, trimmed of all visible fat (¾ pound after trimming)	6 tablespoons cold unsalted fat-free chicken stock
1 tablespoon dry sherry	2 cups broccoli florets
1½ tablespoons oyster sauce	1 tablespoon cornstarch
½ tablespoon low-sodium soy sauce	2 teaspoons peanut or canola oil
½ teaspoon sugar	3 scallions, cut in 1½-inch pieces

1. Slice the meat into 1 × ¼-inch strips.

2. In a bowl combine the sherry, oyster sauce, soy sauce, sugar, and 2 tablespoons of the chicken stock. Add the meat strips and marinate for 5 minutes.

3. Steam the broccoli for 4 minutes, or cook in a microwave on high for 3 minutes.

4. In a separate small bowl, mix the cornstarch with the remaining 4 tablespoons of chicken stock until the mixture is smooth. Drain three-fourths of the meat marinade into this cornstarch mixture.

5. In a wok or 10-inch fry pan heat the oil until sizzling. Add the meat and the remaining marinade to the pan, and stir-fry for 4 minutes, stirring frequently.

6. Add the scallions and broccoli to the beef and cook for 1 more minute. Move the meat, scallions, and broccoli to the sides of the wok or pan, creating a well in the center. Add the cornstarch mixture to the well, and stir as the sauce thickens and clarifies. Serve immediately.

Yield: Serves 4

Each serving has approximately 148 calories, 14.2 g. protein, 6.2 g. total fat (3.7 g. unsaturated fat, 1.8 g. saturated fat), 8.4 g. carbohydrates, 31 mg. cholesterol, 2.5 g. fiber, 316 mg. sodium, 89 mg. calcium.

Exchanges per serving: 2 meat, ¼ starch, 1 vegetable.

Beef with Five-Spice Sauce and Watercress

Chewy beef strips and wilted watercress in a light sauce with warm spices. Look for five-spice powder in oriental markets, spice shops, and the oriental section of supermarkets.

1	teaspoon cornstarch	1	teaspoon five-spice powder
2	tablespoons cold water	1	pound sirloin or beef round,
2	tablespoons low-sodium soy		trimmed of all fat and cut into
	sauce		thin slices (about 1 × ⅛ inch)
½	tablespoon toasted sesame oil	1	teaspoon sugar
2	garlic cloves, finely chopped	2	ounces watercress, stems
1	tablespoon minced ginger		trimmed
3	tablespoons chopped onion		

1. In a small bowl combine the cornstarch, water, and soy sauce until smooth.

2. In a wok or 12-inch fry pan heat the sesame oil, garlic, ginger, onion, and five-spice powder for 1 minute over medium heat. Add the beef, stir-fry for 2 – 3 minutes, stirring frequently. Move the beef away from the center of the pan. Add the cornstarch mixture to the center of the pan, and stir as the mixture thickens. Sprinkle the sugar over the cornstarch, and cook for 20 seconds. Add the watercress, and cook for 45 seconds, until the watercress wilts. Coat the beef and watercress with thickened sauce. Serve immediately.

Yield: Serves 4

Each serving has approximately 184 calories, 22.3 g. protein, 8.4 g. total fat (4.6 g. unsaturated fat, 2.6 g. saturated fat), 3.8 g. carbohydrates, 64 mg. cholesterol, 0.5 g. fiber, 341 mg. sodium, 32 mg. calcium.

Exchanges per serving: 3 meat, ⅒ starch, ½ vegetable.

21 Alarm Chili

The subtle flavor of chocolate and a wallop of chili make this a hearty, pungent, chewy chili. It's even better the next day.

1 pound extra-lean ground beef	3 tablespoons chili powder
1 medium onion, chopped fine	2 tablespoons unsweetened cocoa powder
3 garlic cloves, finely chopped	
1 large green pepper, cut into ½-inch pieces	2 teaspoons sugar
	1 teaspoon crushed hot pepper
2 cans (28-ounce) crushed tomatoes	1 teaspoon Tabasco sauce
	1 can (15-ounce) kidney beans, rinsed in a strainer
2 teaspoons oregano	
2 teaspoons cumin	

1. In a 2½-quart saucepan cook the meat over medium heat until it is well done, about 6–8 minutes, stirring frequently to crumble the meat. Pour off the fat. With a slotted spoon transfer the meat to paper towels to absorb extra fat and wipe the remaining fat residue from the saucepan.

2. In the same pot, sauté the onion, garlic, and green pepper with ½ cup of the crushed tomatoes for 3 minutes. Add the oregano, cumin, chili powder, cocoa powder, sugar, hot pepper, and Tabasco sauce, and continue cooking for 3 minutes more. Add the beans, meat, and the remaining crushed tomatoes, and cook together for 25 minutes over low heat.

Yield: Makes 8 1-cup servings

Each serving has approximately 252 calories, 21.4 g. protein, 8.3 g. total fat (5.9 g. unsaturated fat, 0.5 g. saturated fat), 26.3 g. carbohydrates, 49 mg. cholesterol, 9.2 g. fiber, 358 mg. sodium, 61 mg. calcium.

Exchanges per serving: 3 meat, ¾ starch, 1 vegetable.

Huevos Rancheros

Eggs on a corn tortilla topped with chili, cheese, and herbs.

1 corn tortilla	2 teaspoons fresh cilantro
½ cup 21 Alarm Chili (page 192)	1 tablespoon part-skim
2 egg whites	mozzarella (¼ ounce)
1 scallion, thinly sliced	

1. Steam a tortilla for 10 seconds, or microwave on a plate for 10 seconds, then set it aside. If you don't have a microwave, preheat the broiler.

2. Heat the chili in a small saucepan on top of the stove, or microwave, covered, in a microwave-safe dish on high for 1 minute.

3. Lightly coat a non-stick griddle or fry pan with non-stick cooking spray, and fry the egg whites over medium heat until set.

4. Lay the cooked egg whites over the softened tortilla. Spoon the chili over the egg, and sprinkle the scallion, cilantro, and cheese on top.

5. Place the plate in the microwave and cook on high for 1 minute to melt the cheese, or transfer the prepared tortilla to a baking pan and broil for 1 minute, until the cheese melts.

Yield: Serves 1

Each serving has approximately 211 calories, 18 g. protein, 6 g. total fat (3.3 g. unsaturated fat, 2.2 g. saturated fat), 23 g. carbohydrates, 20.5 mg. cholesterol, 5.7 g. fiber, 165 mg. sodium, 120 mg. calcium. Exchanges per serving: 2 meat, 1 starch, 1 vegetable.

Veal with Peaches, Brandy, and Chervil

Tender meat and sweet fruit in a rich gravy.

1 pound veal scallops	2 tablespoons brandy
3 small fresh peaches	¼ teaspoon salt
2 teaspoons margarine	⅛ teaspoon ground white pepper
1½ cups Basic Chicken Stock (page 86), veal stock, or Beef Stock (page 98)	2 tablespoons chopped fresh chervil
3 tablespoons chopped shallots	

1. Lay the veal on a cutting board, cover with wax paper or plastic wrap, and lightly pound with a mallet to ⅛-inch thickness, being careful not to tear the meat.

2. Peel and slice the peaches, and set aside.

3. Melt 1 teaspoon of the margarine in a 10-inch non-stick fry pan over medium heat. Add half the veal scallops and cook in one layer for 30 seconds per side. Transfer to a warm plate and keep warm in the oven. Melt the remaining margarine in the pan and repeat the procedure for the remaining veal.

4. Add ½ cup of the stock to the pan, and stir to deglaze the pan and incorporate drippings. Add the shallots, brandy, remaining 1 cup of stock, salt, and pepper, and simmer over medium-low heat for 5 minutes. Add the peaches, cook for 2 more minutes, and serve over the veal slices. Garnish with fresh chervil.

Yield: Serves 4

Each serving has approximately 212 calories, 27 g. protein, 5.4 g. total fat (3.5 g. unsaturated fat, 1.6 g. saturated fat), 11.8 g. carbohydrates, 96 mg. cholesterol, 1.4 g. fiber, 240 mg. sodium, 387 mg. calcium. Exchanges per serving: ¾ fruit, 3 meat.

Veal Loaf

Chewy slices of chopped veal to serve hot with Peppery Mushroom Sauce (page 133) or cold, thinly sliced like a pâté, with a dollop of honey mustard.

¼ cup finely chopped onion	2 tablespoons Worcestershire
2 garlic cloves, finely chopped	sauce
¼ pound mushrooms, thinly	½ tablespoon Dijon mustard
sliced	½ tablespoon tomato paste
1 pound extra-lean ground veal	½ teaspoon freshly ground
2 tablespoons fresh bread crumbs	pepper
2 tablespoons wheat germ	

1. Preheat oven to 350° F. Prepare a foil loaf pan 5¾ × 3¼ × 2 inches, by poking 8 holes in the bottom and 2 near the bottom of each side to let the fat run out.

2. In an 8-inch sauté pan, cook the onions, garlic, and mushrooms until softened, about 4 minutes over medium-low heat. Transfer to a bowl and combine with the remaining ingredients.

3. Pack the meat mixture into the loaf pan. Lay the loaf pan on a ridged broiler pan, and bake for 45 minutes.

Yield: Serves 4

Each serving has approximately 253 calories, 40 g. protein, 5.9 g. total fat (3.5 g. unsaturated fat, 1.9 g. saturated fat), 32 g. carbohydrates, 128 mg. cholesterol, 1.4 g. fiber, 229 mg. sodium, 32 mg. calcium. Exchanges per serving: 3½ meat, 1 vegetable.

Veal Parmesan

A low-calorie version of a traditional favorite.

¾ pound veal scallops
2 cups prepared Italian Spaghetti Sauce with Fresh Herbs (page 136)
2 teaspoons olive oil
½ teaspoon freshly ground pepper

4 tablespoons chopped fresh basil or 2 teaspoons dried
1 ounce grated Parmesan cheese
1 ounce grated part-skim mozzarella cheese

1. Preheat broiler.
2. Place the veal between two sheets of plastic wrap or wax paper, and with a wooden mallet lightly pound the veal to a uniform thickness of ⅛ inch.
3. Heat the spaghetti sauce in a small saucepan or microwave in a microwave-safe dish for 2 minutes on high.
4. In a non-stick, 8-inch skillet heat 1 teaspoon of the oil over medium-high heat. Add half the veal slices, sauté for 30 seconds on each side, then transfer them to an 8 × 12-inch bake-and-serve dish. Repeat this procedure with the remaining oil and veal.
5. Sprinkle the pepper and basil over the veal, pour the sauce over, then sprinkle the grated cheeses on top. Broil for 1½ minutes, or until the cheeses melt.

Yield: Serves 4

Each serving has approximately 263 calories, 34.5 g. protein, 10 g. total fat (5.2 g. unsaturated fat, 4 g. saturated fat), 10 g. carbohydrates, 126 mg. cholesterol, 2 g. fiber, 978 mg. sodium, 183 mg. calcium. Exchanges per serving: 4 meat, 1½ vegetable.

Veal Marsala

Tender veal in a full-bodied wine sauce.

1 pound veal scallops
¼ cup unbleached flour
1 teaspoon oil
1 teaspoon margarine
⅓ teaspoon freshly ground pepper
⅓ cup dry marsala wine

⅓ pound sliced mushrooms (2½ cups)
1 cup Basic Chicken Stock (page 86) or veal stock
¼ teaspoon salt
1 tablespoon chopped fresh parsley

1. Place veal between two sheets of wax paper or plastic wrap. With a wooden mallet lightly pound the veal to a uniform thickness of ⅛ inch, being careful not to tear the meat.

2. Pour the flour on a plate or piece of foil or wax paper. Dredge each veal slice in the flour, then shake off any excess. Set the floured veal aside, and discard the remaining flour.

3. In a non-stick 10-inch sauté pan heat ½ teaspoon of the oil and ½ teaspoon of the margarine over medium-high heat until they sizzle. Add half the meat, one layer deep, sprinkle a little pepper on top, and cook for 30 seconds. Turn the veal over and repeat. Transfer the meat to a warmed plate, and repeat the procedure for the rest of the veal.

4. Reduce the heat to medium-low, and to the empty sauté pan add the wine and deglaze the pan by scraping the bottom and sides of the pan as the wine cooks to incorporate the flavorful residue in the sauce. Add the mushrooms and cook for 2–3 minutes. Then add the stock and salt, and cook briskly on high heat for 4–5 minutes to reduce the volume of the sauce by about half.

5. Reduce the heat to medium-low and reheat the veal in the sauce for 1 minute. Serve the veal on warmed plates covered with sauce and garnished with a sprinkling of chopped parsley.

Yield: Serves 4

Each serving has approximately 262 calories, 36.7 g. protein, 7.1 g. total fat (4.6 g. unsaturated fat, 2.1 g. saturated fat), 8 g. carbohydrates, 146 mg. cholesterol, 1 g. fiber, 238 mg. sodium, 17 mg. calcium.

Exchanges per serving: 3½ meat, ½ starch, 1 vegetable.

Marinated Lamb Kabobs

Chewy, moist skewers of lamb with a light herb flavor you can broil or grill.

1⅓ pounds boneless leg of lamb, trimmed of all visible fat (1 pound after trimming)	1 cup Fresh Herb Vinaigrette (page 122)
	4 bamboo or metal skewers

1. Cut the lamb into 1-inch cubes.
2. Pour the vinaigrette into a non-aluminum bowl, add the lamb cubes, cover, and marinate for 2 hours.
3. Preheat the broiler, and place the broiler rack at a middle level.
4. Thread the lamb on the skewer (there will be about 7 pieces per skewer), and broil for 3 minutes on each side.

Yield: Serves 4

Each serving has approximately 193 calories, 24.2 g. protein, 9.7 g. total fat (5.2 g. unsaturated fat, 3.2 g. saturated fat), 1 g. carbohydrates, 79 mg. cholesterol, 0.8 g. fiber, 109 mg. sodium, 15 mg. calcium.

Exchanges per serving: 3 meat.

Lamb and Eggplant Stew

Chewy lamb and eggplant in an unusual stew with the warm flavors of cinnamon, ginger, and coriander.

4 medium garlic cloves, finely chopped	3 tablespoons apple juice concentrate
1 medium onion, chopped	2½ tablespoons lemon juice
2 pounds leg of extra-lean lamb, trimmed of all fat and cut into large chunks (about 1¼ pounds trimmed)	1 teaspoon cinnamon
	1 tablespoon chopped fresh ginger
	1 teaspoon ground coriander
2 cups Beef Stock (page 98)	½ teaspoon salt
1 eggplant, peeled and cut into cubes	½ teaspoon freshly ground black pepper
1 can (6-ounce) tomato paste	2 tablespoons chopped fresh coriander (cilantro)

1. In a 4-quart saucepan, sauté the garlic and onion for 2–3 minutes.

2. Add the lamb chunks and ¼ cup of the beef stock, and cook for 5 minutes over medium heat, stirring occasionally.

3. Add the eggplant and remaining stock, and cook for 5 minutes over medium-low heat.

4. Stir in the tomato paste, apple juice concentrate, lemon juice, cinnamon, ginger, ground coriander, salt, and pepper. Cover and cook on low heat for 15 minutes. Add the fresh coriander, and cook for 5 more minutes.

Yield: Makes 4 1½-cup servings

Each serving has approximately 272 calories, 26.5 g. protein, 7.6 g. total fat (3.3 g. unsaturated fat, 2.8 g. saturated fat), 27 g. carbohydrates, 73.5 mg. cholesterol, 7.6 g. fiber, 361 mg. sodium, 102 mg. calcium.

Exchanges per serving: ⅓ fruit, 3 meat, 3½ vegetable.

Lamb Stew

A hearty country stew with chewy lamb and chunky vegetables in a wine sauce.

1 medium onion, finely chopped	3 celery stalks cut into 1½-inch pieces
4 garlic cloves, finely chopped	1 can (28-ounce) plum tomatoes
2 cups Basic Chicken Stock (page 86)	2 4-inch sprigs fresh rosemary or 2 tablespoons dried
2 pounds extra-lean leg of lamb, trimmed of all visible fat and cut into small cubes (about 1½ pounds trim weight)	½ cup dry red wine or marsala
	1 can (15-ounce) cooked chick-peas, drained
	2 tablespoons chopped fresh parsley
¾ pound potatoes, cubed	¾ teaspoon salt
1¼ pounds butternut squash, seeded and cut into 1½-inch squares	1 teaspoon freshly ground black pepper
1 medium zucchini, cut into 1-inch-thick slices	2 teaspoons fresh thyme or 1 teaspoon dried
1 medium yellow squash, cut into 1-inch-thick slices	3 tablespoons tomato paste

1. In a heavy 6-quart casserole, cook the onion and garlic in 2 tablespoons of the chicken stock for 2 minutes. Add the lamb cubes and ¼ cup of the stock, and cook over low heat for 5 minutes, stirring occasionally.

2. Add the potatoes, butternut squash, zucchini, yellow squash, celery, and the remaining stock, and cook over low heat for 10 minutes, stirring occasionally.

3. Add the tomatoes, rosemary, wine, chick-peas, parsley, salt, pepper, and thyme, then cover the casserole and cook over low heat for 40 minutes.

4. In a 2-cup glass measuring cup mix the tomato paste with ½ cup of the hot broth from the stew until smooth, then pour it back into the stew and stir. Serve.

Yield: Makes 8 2-cup servings

Each serving has approximately 268 calories, 18 g. protein, 5 g. total fat (2.4 g. unsaturated fat, 1.6 g. saturated fat), 37.5 g. carbohydrates, 36 mg. cholesterol, 8 g. fiber, 417 mg. sodium, 120 mg. calcium. Exchanges per serving: 2 meat, 1½ starch, 1 vegetable.

Pork Tenderloin with Fennel and Chestnuts

An unusual combination of sweet pork, licorice-flavored fennel, and nutty chestnuts.

8 fresh chestnuts	1 pound pork tenderloin, trimmed of all visible fat and cut into pieces about 3 inches by 4 inches and ½ inch thick
2½ teaspoons olive oil	
1 garlic clove, finely chopped	
1 ounce fresh fennel root, cut into thin slices about 4 inches by ⅛ inch thick	⅓ teaspoon freshly ground pepper
½ teaspoon salt	
1 cup Basic Chicken Stock (page 86)	

1. Preheat oven to 400° F.

2. Carve an "X" on each chestnut with a small sharp knife. Rub your hands lightly with ½ teaspoon of the oil, then rub the chestnuts in your hands to lightly oil their skins. Place the chestnuts in a baking

pan, and bake for 15 minutes, until the cut skins curl back. Remove the chestnuts from the oven, and peel the skins. Set aside.

3. In a non-stick, 10-inch sauté pan, heat 1 teaspoon of the olive oil. Add the garlic and fennel, and sauté for 2 – 3 minutes, until the fennel is slightly wilted. Add ¼ teaspoon of the salt and the chestnuts, and stir to coat them. Cook for 30 seconds, then transfer all the ingredients to a bowl and set aside.

4. Add ¼ cup of the chicken stock to the sauté pan and stir to pick up the residual juices, then empty the pan into the bowl with the fennel and chestnuts.

5. In the same sauté pan, heat the remaining 1 teaspoon of oil over medium heat. When the pan is hot, add the pork loin pieces, and reduce heat to medium-low. Sprinkle half the pepper over the pork, and cook for 6½ minutes, then turn the pork pieces over, pepper them, and cook for another 6½ minutes. Transfer the cooked meat to a heated serving platter and keep warm.

6. Add the remaining ¾ cup of stock and ¼ teaspoon of salt to the pan, stirring to incorporate any residual juices. Stirring constantly, cook over high heat for 2 minutes to reduce the sauce slightly. Return the fennel-chestnut sauté to the sauce and heat for a minute or two.

7. To serve, spoon some fennel-chestnut sauté and some sauce on top of each tenderloin piece.

Yield: Serves 4

Each serving has approximately 216 calories, 20.7 g. protein, 11.5 g. total fat (7.2 g. unsaturated fat, 3.5 g. saturated fat), 6 g. carbohydrates, 65 mg. cholesterol, 1.5 g. fiber, 319 mg. sodium, 14.4 mg. calcium.

Exchanges per serving: ¾ fat, 3 meat, 1 vegetable.

Pork Tenderloin with Chutney Glaze

A beautiful dish with sweet chewy pork slices under a rich-tasting chutney sauce, and a spinach garnish.

1 teaspoon olive oil	¾ cup Basic Chicken Stock
1 pound lean pork loin slices,	(page 86)
½ inch thick and trimmed of	¼ cup prepared chutney
visible fat	¼ teaspoon salt
⅓ teaspoon freshly ground	4 cups fresh spinach (3½ ounces)
pepper	
1 tablespoon finely chopped	
shallot	

1. In a non-stick 8-inch sauté pan, heat the oil. Add the pork slices, sprinkle half the pepper on top, and cook over low heat for 6½ minutes.

2. Turn the pork over, sprinkle the remaining pepper on top, and cook for 6½ more minutes. Remove the pork from the pan and set aside.

3. Add shallots to the sauté pan, and sauté in remaining pork juices for 1 minute. Slowly add the stock, stirring to deglaze the pan and incorporate the pork juices and residue. Stir in the chutney and salt, and cook over low heat for 2 minutes to reduce the volume of liquid.

4. Meanwhile, steam the spinach for 3 minutes, until lightly wilted, or microwave spinach in a microwave-safe bowl, covered, for 3 minutes on high.

5. Arrange the pork slices on warmed individual dinner plates, and spoon some sauce over each slice. Garnish with cooked spinach, and serve.

Yield: Serves 4

Each serving has approximately 197 calories, 21 g. protein, 10 g. total fat (6 g. unsaturated fat, 3.2 g. saturated fat), 4.8 g. carbohydrates, 64 mg. cholesterol, 1 g. fiber, 205 mg. sodium, 33 mg. calcium.
Exchanges per serving: 3 meat, ⅛ starch, ½ vegetable.

Broiled Ham with Orange Honey Glaze

A zesty orange glaze with a strong mustard flavor over tender ham steaks.

½ tablespoon low-sodium stone-ground mustard
1 tablespoon regular stone-ground mustard
1 tablespoon honey

1 tablespoon orange juice concentrate
¾ pound low-sodium ham steak ½ inch thick, cut into 4 pieces

1. Preheat broiler.
2. In a small bowl combine both stone-ground mustards, honey, and orange juice concentrate.
3. Lay the ham slices on a broiler rack. Brush the glaze over the ham, and broil for 2 minutes on one side only.

Yield: Serves 4

Each serving has approximately 188 calories, 22 g. protein, 5.3 g. total fat (3.3 g. unsaturated fat, 1.6 g. saturated fat), 6.5 g. carbohydrates, 48 mg. cholesterol, 0.1 g. fiber, 845 mg. sodium, 17 mg. calcium. Exchanges per serving: 3 meat, ⅓ starch.

Vegetables

Creamy Country Beets
Broccoli with Anchovies
Sweet and Sour Red Cabbage
Savory Orange Carrots
Cauliflower Puree
Curried Cauliflower with Peas
Baby Corn, Bok Choy, and
   Tofu Stir-Fry
Baked Eggplant with Pesto
Fennel and Chestnuts
Braised Leeks in Red Wine
Double Mushroom Sauté with
   Tarragon
Tomato Okra Sauté
Black-Eyed Peas with
   Tomatoes and Herbs
Sautéed Radicchio and
   Watercress
Three-Pepper Sauté
Creamy Spinach
Spinach Sag Paneer

Spaghetti Squash with Pasta
   Sauce
Butternut Squash with Maple
   Glaze
Turnip Greens with Smoked
   Clams
Hot and Daring Zucchini
   Creole
Zucchini Parmesan
Indian Curried Vegetables
Oriental Vegetable Stir-Fry
Szechuan Stir-Fry
Baked Sweet Potatoes with
   Apples
Almost French-Fried Potatoes
Caraway New Potatoes
Herbed Whole New Potatoes
Mashed Potatoes
Salmon-Stuffed Baked
   Potatoes
Broccoli-Stuffed Potatoes

Creamy Country Beets

Because beets are so healthy and often unsung, we're always trying out new beet recipes. Here's one that's both tangy and creamy.

½ pound beets (about 4 medium)	¼ teaspoon freshly ground
¼ cup plain non-fat yogurt	pepper
1 teaspoon finely sliced green onion or snipped chives	

1. In a 2½-quart pot cook the beets in 6 cups of water at a boil for 45 minutes, or until the beets are fork-tender. Drain in a colander.

Or place the beets in a microwave-safe bowl, add 2 tablespoons of water, cover tightly with plastic wrap, and microwave on high for 10–12 minutes.

2. Cool slightly, then peel and slice the cooked beets, and put them in a serving bowl.

3. Combine the remaining ingredients, and stir into the beets.

Yield: Makes 4 ½-cup servings

Each serving has approximately 23.6 calories, 1.4 g. protein, 0.1 g. total fat (0.02 g. unsaturated fat, 0.02 g. saturated fat), 5 g. carbohydrates, 0.3 mg. cholesterol, 1 g. fiber, 35.3 mg. sodium, 34 mg. calcium.

Exchanges per serving: 1 vegetable.

Broccoli with Anchovies

Crisp broccoli with a hint of garlic and anchovies.

1 pound fresh broccoli	2 garlic cloves, finely chopped
1 can (1½-ounce) anchovies	

1. Cut the broccoli head into florets. Peel the stalks into bite-sized pieces. Steam for 3 minutes, or microwave in a bowl with 2 tablespoons water, covered, for 3 minutes, or just until fork-tender. Drain excess liquid.

2. Drain the anchovies, reserving the oil. Chop enough anchovies to make 1 tablespoon, and set aside.

3. In a 10-inch sauté pan slowly heat 2 teaspoons of the anchovy oil with the garlic until the garlic cooks, about 1 minute.

4. Add the broccoli and chopped anchovies to the pan. Cook for 1 minute on low heat, stirring to mix the ingredients.

Yield: Makes 4 ½-cup servings

Each serving has approximately 57.7 calories, 4.2 g. protein, 2.8 g. total fat (2.2 g. unsaturated fat, 0.4 g. saturated fat), 6.5 g. carbohydrates, 2.5 mg. cholesterol, 3.8 g. fiber, 34.9 mg. sodium, 62 mg. calcium.
Exchanges per serving: ½ fat, 1 vegetable.

Sweet and Sour Red Cabbage

It's sweet, it's sour, it's chewy, it's grainy. It's hard to beat this dish for its variety of superb tastes and textures, not to mention ease of preparation.

4½ cups shredded red cabbage (½ small head)	2 tablespoons red wine vinegar
1 tablespoon brown sugar	½ teaspoon caraway seeds
	¼ teaspoon salt

1. Combine all the ingredients in a heavy, non-aluminum, 2-quart saucepan. Cook over medium-low heat for 10 minutes, covered.

Yield: Makes 4 ½-cup servings

Each serving has approximately 36 calories, 1.2 g. protein, 0.24 g. total fat (0.14 g. unsaturated fat, 0.03 g. saturated fat), 8.7 g. carbohydrates, 0 mg. cholesterol, 1.9 g. fiber, 144 mg. sodium, 46.7 mg. calcium.
Exchanges per serving: 1½ vegetable.

Savory Orange Carrots

Carrot slices with a gentle citrus tang.

¾ pound baby carrots, peeled and cut into 2-inch pieces	1 tablespoon orange juice concentrate or 3 tablespoons orange juice
2 teaspoons chopped fresh thyme or ½ teaspoon dried	2 tablespoons water
	½ teaspoon cornstarch

1. Sprinkle the carrots with thyme. Steam them for 8–10 minutes, until fork-tender, or microwave on high, tightly covered, with 1 tablespoon of water for 7 minutes.

2. Combine the orange juice or concentrate, water, and cornstarch in a small saucepan. Mix until the cornstarch is smooth, then heat until the mixture thickens, or microwave in a glass bowl for 2 minutes on high.

3. Toss the steamed carrots into the sauce and stir to coat.

Yield: Makes 4 ½-cup servings

Each serving has approximately 46.9 calories, 1.1 g. protein, 0.2 g. total fat (0.1 g. unsaturated fat, 0.04 g. saturated fat, 11 g. carbohydrates, 0 mg. cholesterol, 3.1 g. fiber, 56.9 mg. sodium, 31 mg. calcium.
Exchanges per serving: 2 vegetable.

Cauliflower Puree

Thick and creamy, with a dusting of fresh herbs.

4 cups cauliflower florets (from 1 medium head)	⅛ teaspoon white pepper
2½ cups skim milk	2 tablespoons chopped fresh parsley
1½ tablespoons butter-flavored sprinkles	

1. In a heavy 2½-quart saucepan, combine the cauliflower and milk, and cook over low heat for 20 minutes, stirring occasionally so the milk doesn't burn. When the cauliflower is fork-tender, remove from heat.

Or microwave the cauliflower and skim milk, covered tightly, for 12 minutes on high.

2. With a slotted spoon transfer the cauliflower florets to a food processor, and set the remaining milk aside. Puree the cauliflower until smooth, adding about 2 tablespoons of the milk as it purees. Add the butter-flavored sprinkles and the pepper, and puree for 1 minute. The mixture should be thick and creamy like mashed potatoes. If it is too thick, add milk, 1 tablespoon at a time, to reach the desired consistency.

3. Transfer the puree to a warm serving bowl, and garnish with fresh chopped parsley.

Yield: Makes 4 ½-cup servings

Each serving has approximately 46 calories, 3.2 g. protein, 0.3 g. total fat (0.1 g. unsaturated fat, 0 g. saturated fat), 8.9 g. carbohydrates, 0.6 mg. cholesterol, 2.5 g. fiber, 235 mg. sodium, 72 mg. calcium. Exchanges per serving: 2 vegetable.

Curried Cauliflower with Peas

The spirited flavors of curry and red pepper and crisp, colorful vegetables. Low calorie, too.

1 small head cauliflower, outer leaves removed, cut into 1-inch florets	¼ teaspoon ground coriander
	½ pound fresh, raw peas (5 ounces after shelling)
1 teaspoon corn oil	¼ cup unsalted, fat-free chicken or vegetable stock
1 small onion, thinly sliced	
2 small garlic cloves, finely chopped	1½ tablespoons lime juice
½ tablespoon chopped fresh ginger	⅛ teaspoon salt (omit if stock is salted)
½ teaspoon curry powder	⅛ teaspoon crushed red pepper flakes

1. Steam the cauliflower until just tender, about 4–5 minutes. Or microwave with 2 tablespoons water, tightly covered, for 3 minutes on high. Drain.

2. Heat the oil in a 10-inch sauté pan. Add the onion, garlic, ginger, curry, and coriander, and sauté for 2 minutes.

3. Add the cooked cauliflower, peas, stock, lime juice, salt, and crushed red pepper flakes. Cover and cook together for 5 minutes.

Yield: Makes 8 ⅓-cup servings

Each serving has approximately 36.8 calories, 2.1 g. protein, 0.8 g. total fat (0.6 g. unsaturated fat, 0.1 g. saturated fat), 6.3 g. carbohydrates, 0 mg. cholesterol, 2.2 g. fiber, 40.7 mg. sodium, 22.6 mg. calcium.

Exchanges per serving: 1½ vegetable.

Baby Corn, Bok Choy, and Tofu Stir-Fry

Crisp corn and bok choy with soft tofu in a slightly spicy sauce. Ingredients can be found in oriental markets.

2	teaspoons toasted sesame oil	1	can (15-ounce) baby corn
½	tablespoon finely chopped ginger	1	tablespoon dry sherry
		½	tablespoon chili paste with soy bean
1	large garlic clove, finely chopped	1½	tablespoons hoisin sauce
4	cups bok choy, cut diagonally into 1-inch slices	1	tablespoon water
		1	teaspoon cornstarch
¾	pound firm tofu, drained and cut into 1-inch chunks		

1. Heat the oil in a wok or 12-inch fry pan. Add the ginger and garlic, and cook over medium heat for 30 seconds. Add the bok choy, and cook until the leaves soften and turn a deeper green. Add the tofu, baby corn, sherry, chili paste, and hoisin sauce, and cook for 2 minutes on medium heat, stirring frequently.

2. In a small bowl combine the water and cornstarch, stirring until smooth. Move the stir-fry ingredients to the sides of the pan to make a well in the center of the wok or fry pan, and add the cornstarch to the liquid remaining in the well. Stir until the cornstarch clarifies and the mixture thickens. Move the stir-fry ingredients into the well and coat them with this sauce. Serve immediately.

Yield: Makes 8 ½-cup servings

Each serving has approximately 89 calories, 6 g. protein, 3.7 g. total fat (2.7 g. unsaturated fat, 0.5 g. saturated fat), 11.3 g. carbohydrates, 0 mg. cholesterol, 2.6 g. fiber, 80 mg. sodium, 99 mg. calcium.

Exchanges per serving: ¼ fat, ⅜ meat, ⅒ starch, 2 vegetable.

Baked Eggplant with Pesto

Lots of texture in this savory dish — spongy eggplant encased in grainy bread crumbs and topped with basil and chewy cheese.

½ cup bread crumbs	1 recipe Pesto Genovese
½ tablespoon Italian seasoning	(page 132)
½ cup skim milk	2 ounces grated part-skim
1 1-pound eggplant	mozzarella cheese
2 plum tomatoes	

1. Preheat oven to 400° F. Lightly coat a baking sheet with nonstick cooking spray.
2. In a bowl combine the bread crumbs and Italian seasoning, and set aside.
3. Pour the milk into a soup bowl, and set aside.
4. Peel the eggplant, and cut it horizontally into 12 ¾-inch circles. Dip each slice first into the milk, then into the bread crumbs, coating both sides. Lay the eggplant slices on the prepared baking sheet and bake for 25 minutes.
5. Meanwhile, cut the tomatoes into 12 thin slices.
6. When the eggplant slices have finished baking, turn off oven and preheat broiler.
7. Spread ½ tablespoon of pesto over each slice of eggplant, top with a slice of tomato, sprinkle cheese over the tomato slices, and broil for 1½ minutes.

Yield: Makes 12 slices

Each slice has approximately 77 calories, 3.3 g. protein, 4.6 g. total fat (3 g. unsaturated fat, 1.2 g. saturated fat), 7.1 g. carbohydrates, 3.6 mg. cholesterol, 2.1 g. fiber, 189 mg. sodium, 161 mg. calcium. Exchanges per serving: ⅔ fat, ⅙ meat, ⅓ starch, ½ vegetable.

Fennel and Chestnuts

An unusual combination—crisp, roasted chestnuts and the licorice flavor of fennel.

3 ounces chestnuts	⅓ cup unsalted, fat-free chicken stock
1¾ teaspoon olive oil	¼ teaspoon salt
1 garlic clove, minced	
¼ pound fennel, cut into thin strips	

1. Preheat oven to 400° F.
2. To roast the chestnuts, cut an "X" on each chestnut with a small sharp knife. Rub your hands lightly with ¾ teaspoon of the oil, then toss the chestnuts in your hands to lightly oil each shell. Place the chestnuts on a baking pan, and bake until the cut skins curl back, about 15 minutes. Handling the hot chestnuts carefully, peel and lightly chop them.
3. Heat the remaining teaspoon of olive oil in a non-stick 8-inch pan. Add the garlic and fennel and cook together for 5 minutes over medium-low heat, adding 1 or 2 tablespoons of chicken stock, if necessary.
4. Add the chopped chestnuts, salt, and the remaining stock, and cook for 1 more minute over low heat.

Yield: Makes 4 ⅓-cup servings

Each serving has approximately 68 calories, 1 g. protein, 1.6 g. total fat (1.3 g. unsaturated fat, 0.3 g. saturated fat), 12.5 g. carbohydrates, 0 mg. cholesterol, 3.2 g. fiber, 159 mg. sodium, 19 mg. calcium. Exchanges per serving: ¼ fat, 2 vegetable.

Braised Leeks in Red Wine

Sweet and chewy, a lovely accompaniment for fish or a roast.

4 medium leeks	1 tablespoon Parmesan cheese
1¼ cups dry red wine	¼ teaspoon freshly ground black pepper
1 cup water	

1. Trim the root and green stalk from the leeks. Cut the remaining white section in half lengthwise, and wash it carefully to remove dirt between the layers. Slice each half lengthwise again so you have four long quarters.

2. In a non-aluminum 2-quart saucepan bring the red wine and water to a simmer, add the leeks, and cook, covered, for 10 minutes.

3. With a slotted spoon transfer the braised leeks to a warm serving plate, and sprinkle with Parmesan cheese and pepper.

Yield: Serves 4

Each serving has approximately 79 calories, 2 g. protein, 0.6 g. total fat (0.5 g. unsaturated fat, 0.1 g. saturated fat), 12.7 g. carbohydrates, 1 mg. cholesterol, 2 g. fiber, 42 mg. sodium, 71 mg. calcium.
Exchanges per serving: ¼ starch, 2 vegetable.

Double Mushroom Sauté with Tarragon

The chewiness of two types of mushrooms with the subtle flavor of tarragon.

¼ **pound regular button mush-**
  rooms, sliced
¼ **pound fresh shiitake mush-**
  rooms, sliced
1 **teaspoon low-sodium soy sauce**

⅛ **teaspoon freshly ground**
  pepper
2 **teaspoons fresh tarragon or**
  1 teaspoon dried

1. In a heavy-gauge sauté pan, heat the mushrooms over medium heat until they begin to give off their liquid.

2. Add the soy sauce and sauté for 3–4 minutes more. The mushrooms should be tender and moist.

3. Season with ground pepper and tarragon.

Yield: Makes 4 ⅓-cup servings

Each serving has approximately 23.8 calories, 1.1 g. protein, 0.2 g. total fat (0.1 g. unsaturated fat, 0.03 g. saturated fat), 5.5 g. carbohydrates, 0 mg. cholesterol, 1.6 g. fiber, 52.3 mg. sodium, 3.5 mg. calcium.
Exchanges per serving: 1 vegetable.

Tomato Okra Sauté

A colorful trio of spicy, chewy vegetables.

10 ounces fresh baby okra or 1
package (10-ounce) frozen
3 medium plum tomatoes,
seeded and coarsely chopped,
or 1⅓ cup canned whole plum
tomatoes

½ cup fresh corn kernels or
frozen corn, defrosted
1 tablespoon fresh chopped
basil or 1 teaspoon dried
¼ teaspoon freshly ground black
pepper

1. To defrost the okra, boil for 3 minutes in 1 quart of water or microwave on high, covered, for 3 minutes. Or simmer fresh whole okra in 1½ cups of water in a pot, covered, for 8 minutes. Drain in a colander.

2. In a 10-inch sauté pan, heat the tomatoes. Add the okra, corn, basil, and pepper. Cook together for 5 minutes over medium-low heat.

Yield: Makes 4 ½-cup servings

Each serving has approximately 55 calories, 3 g. protein, 0.6 g. total fat (0.3 g. unsaturated fat, 0.1 g. saturated fat), 12.3 g. carbohydrates, 0 mg. cholesterol, 3.3 g. fiber, 136 mg. sodium, 69 mg. calcium. Exchanges per serving: 2 vegetable.

Black-Eyed Peas with Tomatoes and Herbs

A Southern-style stew, with a definite ham flavor.

⅔ cup black-eyed peas
3 cups water
2 ounces turkey ham, finely
diced
3 garlic cloves, finely chopped
3 fresh plum tomatoes, seeded
and chopped
1 teaspoon olive oil
1 teaspoon chopped fresh
rosemary or ½ teaspoon dried

1 teaspoon chopped fresh sage
leaves or ¼ teaspoon ground
⅓ teaspoon freshly ground
pepper
½ cup unsalted, fat-free chicken
or vegetable broth, or reserved
pea broth
1 tablespoon chopped fresh
parsley

1. Wash the peas and pick out any dirt and pebbles. Soak in 3 cups of water overnight, or bring 3 cups of water to a boil, cook the peas for 1 minute, and let soak for 1 hour. Drain.

2. In a large pot bring 6 cups of water to a boil, add the soaked and drained peas, and simmer for 35 minutes, uncovered. Drain and reserve ½ cup of the pea broth.

3. In a 2-quart saucepan, sauté the turkey ham, garlic, and tomatoes in the olive oil for 2 minutes. Add the rosemary, sage, and pepper, and sauté for 2 additional minutes.

4. Add the beans with ½ cup of the cooking broth or stock, and the parsley. Simmer, covered, for 10 minutes.

Yield: Makes 4 ½-cup servings
Each serving has approximately 116 calories, 8.6 g. protein, 2.6 g. total fat (1.6 g. unsaturated fat, 0.6 g. saturated fat), 16 g. carbohydrates, 7.9 mg. cholesterol, 5.9 g. fiber, 147 mg. sodium, 32 mg. calcium. Exchanges per serving: ½ meat, 1 starch, 1 vegetable.

Sautéed Radicchio and Watercress

The flavor in this unusual dish comes from the slightly bitter taste of radicchio, a small, red, Italian lettuce, the peppery watercress, and the faintly sweet and sour sauce; the chewy texture is from the wilted greens.

2 teaspoons margarine	2 heads radicchio lettuce, roots
1 tablespoon orange juice concentrate	removed, leaves torn in half
	2 cups watercress, heavy roots
1 tablespoon red wine vinegar	removed
1 teaspoon low-sodium soy sauce	

1. Melt the margarine in a 10-inch skillet. Stir in the orange juice concentrate, vinegar, and soy sauce. Add the radicchio and watercress, cooking over medium heat until the leaves wilt.

Yield: Makes 4 ½-cup servings
Each serving has approximately 54 calories, 4.3 g. protein, 2.3 g. total fat (1.6 g. unsaturated fat, 0.4 g. saturated fat), 6.2 g. carbohydrates, 0 mg. cholesterol, 4.4 g. fiber, 125 mg. sodium, 175 mg. calcium. Exchanges per serving: ½ fat, 1 vegetable.

Three-Pepper Sauté

A rainbow of bell peppers makes a sweet, crunchy, colorful, and amazingly low-calorie dish.

1 small yellow bell pepper, seeded and cut into thin strips	2 garlic cloves, finely chopped
1 red bell pepper, seeded and cut into thin strips	1 tablespoon Worcestershire sauce
1 green bell pepper, seeded and cut into thin strips	1 tablespoon water
1 red onion, peeled and thinly sliced	1 teaspoon margarine
	¼ teaspoon freshly ground pepper

1. In a 10-inch non-stick sauté pan cook the three peppers, onions, and garlic for 4 minutes without any liquid or fat. Add the Worcestershire sauce and water, and cook over medium heat for 2 minutes, or to desired tenderness, stirring frequently. If you need more liquid, add water, a tablespoon at a time.

2. Add the margarine and ground pepper, and stir to coat the vegetables lightly.

Yield: Makes 8 ½-cup servings

Each serving has approximately 18.4 calories, 0.05 g. protein, 0.6 g. total fat (0.4 g. unsaturated fat, 0.1 g. saturated fat), 3.1 g. carbohydrates, 0 mg. cholesterol, 0.7 g. fiber, 27.4 mg. sodium, 8.4 mg. calcium.

Exchanges per serving: ⅛ fat, ½ vegetable.

Creamy Spinach

For creamed spinach lovers, a low-calorie version with the salty bite of Parmesan cheese and the colorful crunch of red bell peppers.

1 package (10-ounce) fresh spinach, washed, drained, with thick stems removed, or 1 package (10-ounce) frozen chopped spinach, defrosted and well drained
3 tablespoons finely chopped onion (about ½ small onion)
1 garlic clove, finely chopped
1 tablespoon white wine

1 teaspoon margarine
1 teaspoon unbleached flour
½ cup skim milk
2 tablespoons Parmesan cheese
⅛ teaspoon freshly ground pepper
¼ teaspoon salt
2 tablespoons finely chopped red bell peppers

1. Steam fresh spinach for 5 – 7 minutes, or microwave, uncovered, on high for 4 minutes. Squeeze excess water from the spinach, chop coarsely, and set aside. Defrosted spinach needs no cooking.

2. In a 2-quart saucepan, heat the chopped onion and garlic in the wine for 1 minute, until the wine evaporates. Add the margarine, let melt, then sprinkle in the flour. Stir to incorporate the flour, and cook over low heat for 1 minute, stirring continuously to avoid burning the flour. Slowly add the milk, stirring as the sauce thickens. Season with Parmesan cheese, pepper, and salt.

3. Stir in the spinach and chopped red pepper, and cook for a few minutes to heat the vegetables.

Yield: Makes 4 ⅓-cup servings

Each serving has approximately 55 calories, 4.4 g. protein, 2.1 g. total fat (1.1 g. unsaturated fat, 0.8 g. saturated fat), 5.5 g. carbohydrates, 2.3 mg. cholesterol, 2.6 g. fiber, 264 mg. sodium, 148 mg. calcium. Exchanges per serving: ¼ meat, 1½ vegetable.

Spinach Sag Paneer

This curried creamy spinach dish is traditional in India. We substituted feta, which is widely available, for the traditional Indian cheese. Try it with Tandoori Chicken (page 168).

2 small garlic cloves, chopped	1 package (10-ounce) fresh
½ tablespoon chopped fresh	spinach, washed, drained,
ginger	with thick stems removed, or
½ medium onion, chopped	1 package (10-ounce) frozen
½ teaspoon curry powder	whole spinach, defrosted and
1 teaspoon corn or safflower oil	well drained
	1 ounce feta cheese

1. In a 10-inch sauté pan, cook the garlic, ginger, onion, and curry powder in the oil over medium heat for 2 to 3 minutes.

2. Add the spinach and stir. When the spinach begins to wilt, crumble in the feta cheese, and continue stirring until the cheese melts. Remove from heat and serve.

Yield: Makes 4 ½-cup servings

Each serving has approximately 58.2 calories, 3.6 g. protein, 3.1 g. total fat (1.5 g. unsaturated fat, 1.3 g. saturated fat), 5.8 g. carbohydrates, 6.2 mg. cholesterol, 3. g. fiber, 136 mg. sodium, 116 mg. calcium.

Exchanges per serving: ¼ medium-fat meat, 1¼ vegetable.

Spaghetti Squash with Pasta Sauce

Juicy strands of squash bathed in a tangy basil tomato sauce.

2½ pound spaghetti squash	¼ teaspoon freshly ground
2 cups Italian Spaghetti Sauce	pepper
with Fresh Herbs (page 136)	2 tablespoons grated Parmesan
¼ cup fresh basil leaves,	cheese
shredded, or 2 teaspoons	
dried basil	

1. Preheat oven to 350° F. if baking the squash.

2. Cut the squash in half crosswise. Cook according to either method:

In oven: Place the squash halves cut side down in a baking pan. Bake for 50–60 minutes, or until the squash is easily pierced with a sharp knife.

In microwave: Place the squash cut side down in a microwave-safe dish with ¼ cup of water, and cover tightly with plastic wrap. Cook on high for 10 minutes.

3. Meanwhile, heat the spaghetti sauce, basil, and pepper in a saucepan on top of the stove over low heat for about 10 minutes.

4. With a fork carefully remove the hot squash meat; it will come out in spaghetti-like strands. Put it on a warm serving platter, pour over the hot sauce, and sprinkle the top with the Parmesan cheese.

Yield: Serves 4

Each serving has approximately 138 calories, 4.8 g. protein, 2.6 g. total fat (1.4 g. unsaturated fat, 0.8 g. saturated fat), 27 g. carbohydrates, 2 mg. cholesterol, 10.5 g. fiber, 217 mg. sodium, 129 mg. calcium. Exchanges per serving: ¼ meat, 2 starch, 2 vegetable.

Butternut Squash with Maple Glaze

Baking brings out the full sweetness of the squash and glaze, but if you're pressed for time, the microwave can definitely do the job.

2 pound butternut squash	4 teaspoons low-calorie maple
2 teaspoons margarine	syrup

1. Preheat the oven to 400° F. if baking the squash.

2. Cut the squash in half and remove the seeds. Cut each half into eight pieces, each about 2½ to 3 inches square. Place them in one layer in an oven-proof glass or ceramic serving dish, skin-side down.

3. Heat the margarine and syrup together on the range, or microwave on high for 30 seconds.

4. Brush or spoon the hot maple mixture over the squash sections. Cook according to either method:

In oven: Cover the baking dish with foil, then bake for 1 hour. Test for tenderness with a fork.

In microwave: Cover the dish with plastic wrap, and cook on high for 8 minutes. Rotate the dish 180 degrees and microwave for 8 more minutes. Test for tenderness with a fork. If necessary, recover, rotate dish again, and microwave for an additional 2 to 4 minutes.

5. Remove from oven and uncover. Spoon any maple sauce from the pan over the top of the squash.

Yield: Serves 8

Each serving has approximately 57 calories, 1 g. protein, 1 g. total fat (0.8 g. unsaturated fat, 0.2 g. saturated fat), 12.6 g. carbohydrates, 0 mg. cholesterol, 3.2 g. fiber, 19 mg. sodium, 46.6 mg. calcium. Exchanges per serving: ⅛ fat, ⅔ starch.

Turnip Greens with Smoked Clams

Turnip greens are one of a variety of pot greens well known in the South. To their slightly bitter, al dente texture, we've added the piquant flavor of smoked clams.

1 **bunch young turnip greens** (¾ pound)	1 **can (3.66-ounce) smoked clams, including juices**

1. Wash the turnip greens carefully, trim stems, and drain in a colander.

2. Steam the turnip greens in a covered 3- to 4-quart pot for 10 minutes. Test for doneness. If you like your greens softer, continue cooking for several more minutes.

3. Meanwhile, drain the clams over a bowl and reserve the liquid. Rinse the drained clams under water to eliminate excess salt and oil, and pick out any shell fragments.

4. In a 10-inch cast-iron pan, heat 2 teaspoons of the clam liquid. Add the cooked greens, sauté for 2 minutes over medium-high heat. Add the drained clams and cook for 1 more minute.

Yield: Makes 4 ¾-cup servings

Each serving has approximately 55 calories, 7.6 g. protein, 0.7 g. total fat (0.3 g. unsaturated fat, 0.1 g. saturated fat), 5.04 g. carbohydrates, 17.3 mg. cholesterol, 2.6 g. fiber, 53.2 mg. sodium, 141 mg. calcium. Exchanges per serving: ¾ meat, ¾ vegetable.

Hot and Daring Zucchini Creole

Spicy, spicy, spicy. You could call it 21 alarm zucchini.

⅓ cup finely chopped onion	¼ teaspoon Tabasco
2 garlic cloves, finely chopped	½ teaspoon prepared mustard
⅓ cup low-sodium tomato juice	⅛ teaspoon crushed red peppers
1 pound zucchini, sliced in ¼-inch rounds	2 teaspoons grated Parmesan cheese
2 plum tomatoes, cored and finely chopped	

1. Combine the onion, garlic, and 2 tablespoons of the tomato juice in a heavy skillet. Cook on medium heat for 2 minutes, stirring frequently.

2. Add the remaining tomato juice, zucchini slices, tomatoes, Tabasco, mustard, and red peppers, and cook on medium-low heat, stirring frequently, for 3–4 minutes, or until the zucchini is tender but still firm.

3. Sprinkle the cheese on top, stir, and cook for 1 more minute.

Yield: Makes 4 ½-cup servings

Each serving has approximately 36 calories, 2.3 g. protein, 0.6 g. total fat, (0.2 g. unsaturated fat, 0.2 g. saturated fat) 6.7 g. carbohydrates, 0.6 mg. cholesterol, 2 g. fiber, 31 mg. sodium, 39 mg. calcium. Exchanges per serving: 1½ vegetable.

Zucchini Parmesan

Al dente zucchini rounds and tender chunks of tomato in light basil-flavored tomato juices, with the lively bite of Parmesan cheese.

¾ pound zucchini (about
2 medium)

3 plum tomatoes, seeded and chopped, or 1¼ cups canned crushed tomatoes

1 tablespoon fresh chopped basil or 1 teaspoon dried (omit if using canned tomatoes that include basil)

2 tablespoons grated Parmesan cheese

1. Preheat broiler.
2. Cut the zucchini into ¼-inch diagonal slices, and steam just until fork-tender, about 5 minutes. Or cook in microwave on high for 3 minutes, covered.
3. Layer the zucchini and tomatoes in an 8-inch round or square bake-and-serve dish, sprinkle with crushed basil, top with Parmesan cheese, and broil for 3 minutes, or until the cheese melts.

Yield: Makes 4 ⅔-cup servings
Each serving has approximately 36 calories, 2.6 g. protein, 1 g. total fat (0.4 g. unsaturated fat, 0.6 g. saturated fat), 5.2 g. carbohydrates, 2 mg. cholesterol, 1.8 g. fiber, 54 mg. sodium, 60 mg. calcium.
Exchanges per serving: ¼ meat, 1 vegetable.

Indian Curried Vegetables

Colorful crisp fresh vegetables in a spicy curry sauce.

1 tablespoon corn oil

2 garlic cloves, peeled and chopped

1 slice fresh ginger cut 1 inch square and ⅛ inch thick

2 teaspoons curry powder

1 medium onion, sliced thin

3 medium carrots, peeled and sliced ¼ inch thick

1½ cups fresh string beans, ends trimmed

2 tablespoons sherry or white wine

½ green bell pepper, seeded and cut into 1-inch squares

1 red or yellow bell pepper, seeded and cut into 1-inch squares

2 tablespoons water

3 cups fresh spinach (about 6 ounces), washed and drained

2 tablespoons raisins

Sauce:

2 tablespoons lemon juice

1 tablespoon low-sodium soy sauce

2 tablespoons orange juice

2 tablespoons water

1 teaspoon cornstarch

1. Heat the oil in a wok or 12-inch sauté pan. Add the garlic, ginger, curry powder, and onion. Sauté for 2 minutes.

2. Add the carrots and cook for 2 minutes, stirring frequently over medium heat. Add the string beans and the sherry or wine, and sauté for 2 minutes, stirring frequently. Add the bell peppers and 2 tablespoons of water, and cook for 2 more minutes. Discard the ginger slice.

3. Add the spinach and the raisins to the pan, and sauté for 2 minutes, or until the spinach wilts. Move all the vegetables to one side of the pan.

4. In a separate bowl combine the sauce ingredients and stir until free of lumps. Add to the pan, stirring the sauce as it thickens. When the sauce is thick, combine it with the vegetables.

Yield: Makes 8 ½-cup servings

Each serving has approximately 63 calories, 2 g. protein, 2 g. total fat (1.6 g. unsaturated fat, 0.3 g. saturated fat), 10.4 g. carbohydrates, 0 mg. cholesterol, 2.8 g. fiber, 104 mg. sodium, 47.8 mg. calcium. Exchanges per serving: ⅓ fat, 2 vegetable.

Oriental Vegetable Stir-Fry

This is a mélange of crisp fresh oriental vegetables in a mild sauce. Napa is a light green, long, curly cabbage; seitan, also called braised mock-meat, is made of gluten, a protein found in wheat, and has a chewy, chicken-like texture. If you can't find seitan, substitute tofu. The exotic ingredients are available in oriental stores and many supermarkets.

1 teaspoon toasted sesame oil
1 teaspoon chopped fresh ginger
1 garlic clove, finely chopped
1 medium carrot, peeled and cut into ¼-inch slices
8 cups napa cabbage, stems and leaves, cut into 1-inch slices
1 tablespoon dry sherry

1 can (10-ounce) seitan (also called braised mock-meat), rinsed in a colander
1 teaspoon oyster sauce
1 teaspoon low-sodium soy sauce
½ tablespoon water
1 teaspoon cornstarch

1. Heat the oil in a wok or 12-inch fry pan, then add the ginger and garlic, and cook for 30 seconds over medium heat.

2. Add the carrot, and stir-fry for 1 minute. Add the napa and sherry, and cook for 3 – 4 minutes, until stems soften slightly. Add the seitan, and stir-fry for 2 minutes.

3. Meanwhile, in a small bowl combine the oyster sauce, soy sauce, water, and cornstarch, and stir until smooth.

4. Move the stir-fry ingredients to the sides of the pan, leaving a well in the center. Add the soy mixture to the well, and cook for 1 minute, or until sauce thickens. Move the vegetables into the well to coat them with the sauce. Serve immediately.

Yield: Makes 4 1-cup servings
Each serving has approximately 48 calories, 4.3 g. protein, 1.5 g. total fat (1.1 g. unsaturated fat, 0.1 g. saturated fat), 5.3 g. carbohydrates, 0 mg. cholesterol, 2 g. fiber, 54 mg. sodium, 41 mg. calcium.
Exchanges per serving: ¼ fat, 1½ vegetable.

Szechuan Stir-Fry

Colorful crunchy fresh vegetables in a very hot and very spicy sauce.

1 tablespoon sherry	½ teaspoon crushed red pepper flakes
2 tablespoons low-sodium soy sauce	
1 teaspoon sugar	4 ounces asparagus, cut in 1-inch pieces (about 8 stalks)
1 tablespoon Szechuan seasoning	½ large red bell pepper, cut into ¼ × 2-inch pieces
1 tablespoon cornstarch	1 ounce snow peas, ends trimmed
¼ cup cold, unsalted, fat-free chicken stock, vegetable stock, or water	3½ ounces shiitake mushrooms, stems trimmed, each mushroom cut in half
½ tablespoon toasted sesame oil	
1 teaspoon finely chopped ginger root	1 can (8-ounce) water chestnuts, drained
2 garlic cloves, finely chopped	2 scallions, thinly sliced

1. In a small bowl combine the sherry, soy sauce, sugar, Szechuan seasoning, cornstarch, and stock, and stir until smooth. Set aside.

2. In a wok or 12-inch fry pan, heat the oil, ginger, garlic, and red pepper flakes over medium heat. Do not let the oil smoke.

3. Add the asparagus pieces, and stir-fry for 2 minutes, then move the asparagus to the sides of the pan. Add the bell pepper and snow peas in the center, cook for 1 minute, and move them to the sides of the pan. Add the mushrooms to the center of the pan, cook for 1 minute, then add the water chestnuts and cook for 1 minute.

4. Move all the vegetables to the sides of the pan, making a well in the center. Stir the cornstarch mixture again, then pour it into the well, stirring as the mixture thickens.

5. Add the scallions, and stir to coat the vegetables with the sauce. Serve immediately.

Yield: Makes 8 ½-cup servings
Each serving has approximately 49 calories, 1.5 g. protein, 1 g. total fat (0.8 g. unsaturated fat, 0.2 g. saturated fat), 9 g. carbohydrates, 0 mg. cholesterol, 1.6 g. fiber, 154 mg. sodium, 13 mg. calcium.
Exchanges per serving: ⅙ fat, ⅙ starch, 1 vegetable.

Baked Sweet Potatoes with Apples

Warmly spiced chunks of apples folded into sweet, creamy potatoes.

2 small sweet potatoes or yams (about 10 ounces total)	¼ teaspoon nutmeg
2 tablespoons skim milk	⅓ teaspoon cinnamon
½ medium Granny Smith or Rome apple	

1. Preheat oven to 425° F.
2. Pierce the sweet potatoes with a fork, and bake until soft to the touch, about 50 minutes, or microwave on high, uncovered, for 11–13 minutes. Let the potatoes cool.
3. Cut the potatoes in half and carefully scoop out the filling.
4. Transfer the filling to a bowl, and beat with an electric beater until smooth, adding a tablespoon of milk at a time. Set aside.
5. Peel and chop the apple, and sprinkle with nutmeg and cinnamon. Microwave in a bowl for 15 seconds, or heat in a saucepan for 5 minutes with 1 tablespoon of water to soften slightly.
6. Fold the apples into the sweet potato, and bake for 10 minutes at 425° or microwave for 2 minutes on high.

Yield: Makes 4 ⅓-cup servings

Each serving has approximately 86 calories, 1.5 g. protein, 0.2 g. total fat (0.1 g. unsaturated fat, 0.1 g. saturated fat), 20.2 g. carbohydrates, 0.1 mg. cholesterol, 2.5 g. fiber, 11.5 mg. sodium, 32 mg. calcium. Exchanges per serving: 1 starch.

Almost French-Fried Potatoes

Here is a crisp version of a great American favorite, with all the traditional flavor and a lot fewer calories and fat.

1 pound baking potatoes (about 2 or 3 medium size)	2–3 teaspoons onion powder, garlic powder, chili powder or paprika
½ tablespoon corn oil	

1. Preheat oven to 450° F.
2. Peel the potatoes and cut into ¼ × ¼ × 3-inch strips.

3. Pour the oil into a wide 1- or 2-quart bowl. Toss the potato strips in the oil. Shake off any excess oil, then place the strips on an un-greased baking pan. Sprinkle them with onion powder or one of the other seasonings.

4. Bake for 20 minutes, or until one side of the potato strips are brown. Turn them over and bake until brown and crisp on the other side, about 10 more minutes.

5. Drain on absorbent paper towels.

Yield: Makes 50–60 fries and serves 6

Each serving has approximately 84 calories, 1.6 g. protein, 1.2 g. total fat (1 g. unsaturated fat, 0.2 g. saturated fat), 17.4 g. carbohydrates, 0 mg. cholesterol, 1.2 g. fiber, 4.3 mg. sodium, 7 mg. calcium. Exchanges per serving: ¼ fat, 1 starch.

Caraway New Potatoes

Caraway seeds provide the snappy anise taste and the grainy texture.

12 small red or white new potatoes (about 1 pound)	1 teaspoon caraway seeds
½ tablespoon corn oil	¼ teaspoon salt

1. Place the potatoes in a 2-quart pot with enough water to cover them. Bring to a boil, then simmer, covered, until fork-tender, about 15–18 minutes, depending on the size of the potatoes. Drain the cooked potatoes in a colander.

Or microwave the potatoes with 2 tablespoons of water in a microwave-safe dish, tightly covered, for 10 minutes on high. Drain.

2. In a 10-inch cast-iron pan, heat the oil on low. Add the caraway seeds and salt, then stir in the potatoes until they are well coated.

Yield: Serves 4

Each serving has approximately 116 calories, 2.2 g. protein, 1.9 g. total fat (1.5 g. unsaturated fat, 0.3 g. saturated fat), 23.1 g. carbohydrates, 0 mg. cholesterol, 1.8 g. fiber, 138 mg. sodium, 10.5 mg. calcium. Exchanges per serving: ½ fat, 1¼ starch.

Herbed Whole New Potatoes

The bite of garlic and the piquant flavor of herbs enliven the tender texture of new potatoes.

12	small white or red new potatoes (about 1 pound)	2	tablespoons fresh basil, thyme, or parsley, finely chopped
1	teaspoon margarine	⅛	teaspoon salt
2	garlic cloves, finely chopped		

1. Place the potatoes in a 2-quart pot with enough water to cover them. Bring to a boil, then simmer, covered, until fork-tender, about 15–18 minutes, depending on the size of the potatoes. Drain the cooked potatoes in a colander.

Or microwave the potatoes with 2 tablespoons of water in a microwave-safe dish, tightly covered, for 10 minutes on high. Drain.

2. In an 8- or 10-inch non-stick sauté pan melt the margarine over medium heat. Add the garlic, herbs, and salt, then the potatoes. Cook over low heat for another minute, stirring to coat the potatoes with the seasonings.

Yield: Serves 4

Each serving has approximately 115 calories, 2.6 g. protein, 1.2 g. total fat (0.8 g. unsaturated fat, 0.2 g. saturated fat), 24.7 g. carbohydrates, 0 mg. cholesterol, 2.1 g. fiber, 84 mg. sodium, 56.8 mg. calcium. Exchanges per serving: ¼ fat, 1 starch, ½ vegetable.

Mashed Potatoes

Creamy, creamy, creamy — that's the texture of these fluffy, buttery-tasting potatoes.

1½	pounds Idaho potatoes, cut into sixths	¼	teaspoon salt
⅓	cup skim milk	¼	teaspoon white pepper
1½	tablespoons butter-flavored sprinkles		

1. Bring 2 quarts of water to a boil in a 4-quart pot. Add potato chunks and boil for 15–20 minutes, or until fork-tender. Drain in a

colander, then rinse with cold water. Peel the potatoes and place them in a medium-sized bowl.

2. Using a hand-held potato masher or an electric beater, mash the boiled potatoes. Slowly add the milk, butter-flavored sprinkles, salt, and pepper, and stir vigorously until fluffy.

Yield: Makes 8 ½-cup servings

Each serving has approximately 81.7 calories, 2.3 g. protein, 0.1 g. total fat (0.05 g. unsaturated fat, 0.05 g. saturated fat), 18.2 g. carbohydrates, 0.3 mg. cholesterol, 1.3 g. fiber, 80.8 mg. sodium, 30 mg. calcium.

Exchanges per serving: 1 starch.

Salmon-Stuffed Baked Potatoes

Creamy potatoes, flecked with peas, bits of smoked salmon, nuggets of crisp celery, and snippets of fragrant dill.

2 **baking potatoes (about 1 pound total)**	½ **tablespoon snipped fresh dill or ½ teaspoon dried dill**
⅓ **cup skim milk**	1½ **tablespoons finely chopped nova lox (about 1 ounce)**
¼ **teaspoon ground black pepper**	¼ **cup finely chopped celery**
¼ **teaspoon salt**	
¼ **cup frozen peas, defrosted**	

1. Prick the potatoes with a fork, and bake in oven for 1 hour at 450°, or microwave, uncovered, on high for 11–13 minutes. Let the potatoes cool. Reduce oven temperature to 350°.

2. Cut the potatoes in half lengthwise. Carefully scoop out the filling, leaving the skins intact. In a bowl mash the potatoes by hand or with an electric beater. Add half the milk, the pepper, and salt. Continue beating to puree the potatoes, adding the rest of the milk, a little at a time. With a rubber spatula, carefully fold in the peas, dill, nova lox, and celery.

3. Divide the filling among the potato skins. Reheat for 20 minutes in the oven, or microwave, uncovered, for 3 minutes on high.

4. Meanwhile, preheat the broiler. When the potatoes are hot, place them under the broiler until their tops are lightly brown, about 3–4 minutes.

Yield: Serves 4

Each serving has approximately 148 calories, 5.2 g. protein, 0.5 g. total fat (0.3 g. unsaturated fat, 0.1 g. saturated fat), 31.4 g. carbohydrates, 2 mg. cholesterol, 3.3 g. fiber, 216 mg. sodium, 45.4 mg. calcium. Exchanges per serving: 1¾ starch.

Broccoli-Stuffed Potatoes

A creamy cheese sauce naps crisp broccoli florets in a baked potato. We like this for supper, with a large salad and fruit. Oh, yes, and we freeze the rest of the cheddar for next time.

2   baking potatoes, about
    1 pound total weight
2   cups broccoli florets (about
    two stalks)

Cheese Sauce:

½   tablespoon margarine
½   tablespoon unbleached flour
¾   cup skim milk
1   ounce sharp cheddar cheese,
    grated
⅛   teaspoon salt
⅛   teaspoon ground white pepper

1.   Pierce the potatoes with a fork, then bake for 1 hour at 475° F. or place on a paper towel and microwave on high for 11–13 minutes, uncovered. Let the potatoes cool for 5 minutes.

2.   Steam the broccoli for 3 minutes or microwave with 1 tablespoon of water, covered, on high for 3 minutes. Drain the broccoli.

3.   In a small saucepan, melt the margarine over medium heat, then sprinkle the flour over the margarine and stir continuously. Cook this flour-margarine mixture for about 2 minutes. Slowly add the milk, stirring with a whisk to prevent lumps as the mixture thickens. Stir in the cheese with a spoon, letting it melt. Season with salt and pepper.

4.   To serve, cut each potato in half lengthwise. Lightly press each half at its ends to loosen the potato meat. Divide the broccoli over each potato half and top with the cheese sauce.

Yield: Serves 4

Each serving has approximately 196 calories, 7.7 g. protein, 4.1 g. total fat (2 g. unsaturated fat, 1.9 g. saturated fat), 34 g. carbohydrates, 8.2 mg. cholesterol, 4.1 g. fiber, 172 mg. sodium, 141 mg. calcium. Exchanges per serving: 1 fat, 1½ starch, 1 vegetable.

Grains and Pasta

Sweet and Crunchy Brown Rice
Brown Rice with Fresh Roasted Chestnuts
Wild and Brown Rice
Cajun Jambalaya Rice
Chinese Fried Rice
Dilled Persian Rice
Bulgur Pilaf with Basil and Pine Nuts
Wild Rice Frittata
Lemon Couscous
Polenta with Pesto
Speckled Kasha
Chinese Noodles with Asparagus

Pasta Tutti
Angel Hair with Scallops and Crabmeat
Fettuccine with Mushroom Stroganoff
Vegetable Lasagna
Lasagna Roll-ups
Pasta Fagioli
Penne with Basil and Sweet Peppers
Linguine and Lobster
Linguine with Tomato Clam Sauce
Spicy Italian "Meatballs" with Spaghetti

Sweet and Crunchy Brown Rice

Currants and chestnuts are the crunchy surprises here.

1 cup brown rice
⅓ cup currants
½ cup canned water chestnuts,
  finely sliced
¼ cup fresh chopped parsley
2 cups plus 2 tablespoons water

1. Rinse the rice in a fine-mesh colander to remove some of the outer starch.
2. In a 1½-quart saucepan, sauté the rice over medium-high heat until the water clinging to the rice has evaporated, stirring occasionally. Add the remaining ingredients and bring to a boil. Reduce heat to low, cover, and cook for 40 minutes.

Yield: Makes 8 ½-cup servings
Each serving has approximately 105 calories, 2.1 g. protein, 0.5 g. fat (0.3 g. unsaturated fat, 0.1 g. saturated fat), 23.5 g. carbohydrates, 0 mg. cholesterol, 1.5 g. fiber, 4 mg. sodium, 15.3 mg. calcium. Exchanges per serving: ½ fruit, 1 starch.

Brown Rice with Fresh Roasted Chestnuts

An unusual combination with lots of crunchy texture.

¼ pound fresh chestnuts
1 teaspoon corn oil
1½ cups water
¾ cup brown rice, rinsed

1. Preheat oven to 400° F.
2. To roast the chestnuts, carve an "X" on each chestnut with a small sharp knife. Rub your hands lightly with the oil, then rub the chestnuts in your hands to lightly oil their skins. Place the chestnuts in a baking pan, and bake for 15 minutes, until the cut skins curl back.

3. Remove the chestnuts from the oven, and peel the skins. Chop the chestnuts into small pieces (don't grind them).

4. Bring the water to a boil. Add the rice and chestnuts. Bring to a second boil, cover, and reduce heat as low as possible. Cook for 45 minutes.

Yield: Makes 8 ⅓-cup servings

Each serving has approximately 90 calories, 1.5 g. protein, 0.5 g. total fat (0.34 g. unsaturated fat, 0.12 g. saturated fat), 19.6 g. carbohydrates, 0 mg. cholesterol, 2.1 g. fiber, 2.1 mg. sodium, 8 mg. calcium. Exchanges per serving: 1 starch.

Wild and Brown Rice

Two rices with many textures—nutty, crunchy, chewy, grainy—flecked with fresh parsley.

1¼ cups water
¼ teaspoon salt
¼ cup brown rice
¼ cup wild rice
¼ cup finely chopped parsley

1. Boil the water and salt in a 1-quart saucepan.

2. Add the two rices and parsley, bring to a boil, then reduce heat to low. Cover and cook for 50 minutes.

Yield: Makes 4 ⅓-cup servings

Each serving has approximately 77 calories, 2.3 g. protein, 0.3 g. total fat (0.2 g. unsaturated fat, 0.1 g. saturated fat), 16.3 g. carbohydrates, 0 mg. cholesterol, 1.5 g. fiber, 137 mg. sodium, 11.3 mg. calcium. Exchanges per serving: 1 starch.

Cajun Jambalaya Rice

The lively pungent flavors and aromas of Cajun cooking, with bites of vegetables and ham-flavored turkey. We like it as a supper entree with a salad and a grainy bread.

1 medium onion, chopped	¼ teaspoon ground white pepper
3 garlic cloves, finely chopped	¼ teaspoon ground black pepper
1 large, green bell pepper, cut into ½-inch pieces	¾ teaspoon red pepper flakes or cayenne pepper
2¼ cups Basic Chicken Stock (page 86)	½ teaspoon cumin
5 scallions, finely sliced	¼ teaspoon allspice
1 cup raw, long-grained brown rice	¼ pound shrimp, peeled and deveined
3 fresh Italian plum tomatoes, cored, seeded, and chopped	dash Tabasco sauce (optional)
¼ pound baked turkey ham, all visible fat removed, cut into ½-inch cubes	¼ cup chopped fresh parsley

1. In an 8-quart pot sauté the onion, garlic, and green pepper in 3 tablespoons of stock for 5 minutes.

2. Add two-thirds of the scallions, the rice, and tomatoes, and cook for 5 minutes over medium-low heat, adding a little more of the stock if necessary.

3. Add the cubed turkey ham, the three peppers, cumin, allspice, and the remaining stock, and cook on very low heat, covered, for 40 minutes. Add the shrimp and cook for 2 minutes.

4. Taste for spiciness. You can add 5–6 drops of Tabasco sauce for a more pungent flavor.

5. Serve garnished with parsley and the remaining scallions.

Yield: Makes 4 1-cup servings

Each serving has approximately 276 calories, 16.4 g. protein, 3.4 g. total fat (1.9 g. unsaturated fat, 0.9 g. saturated fat), 45.7 g. carbohydrates, 59 mg. cholesterol, 4.5 g. fiber, 331 mg. sodium, 67 mg. calcium.

Exchanges per serving: 1 meat, 2½ starch, 1 vegetable.

Chinese Fried Rice

Lots of crunch from scallions, ham-flavored turkey slivers, and peas in rice, cooked the Chinese way.

2⅓ cups cooked brown rice, cold	¼ cup frozen peas, defrosted
1 tablespoon corn oil	3 tablespoons finely chopped scallions (about 3 scallions)
2 egg whites, lightly beaten	
½ ounce lean turkey ham, cut into fine slivers (about one slice)	1½ tablespoons low-sodium soy sauce
	¼ teaspoon black pepper

1. Separate the rice with a fork. Add a tablespoon or two of water if necessary to moisten and separate. Set aside.

2. Heat the oil in a wok or fry pan. Add the lightly beaten egg whites, ham, and peas, and cook on medium heat for 1 minute. Add the rice, and stir to combine the ingredients. Add the scallions, soy sauce, and pepper, and cook for 1 more minute.

Yield: Makes 8 ⅓-cup servings

Each serving has approximately 95.6 calories, 3.1 g. protein, 2.2 g. total fat (1.7 g. unsaturated fat, 0.34 g. saturated fat), 15.8 g. carbohydrates, 0.1 mg. cholesterol, 1.3 g. fiber, 142 mg. sodium, 13.6 mg. calcium.

Exchanges per serving: ½ fat, 1 starch.

Dilled Persian Rice

Basmati is a Middle Eastern and Indian rice with a wonderful buttery aroma. It is available in specialty or health food stores. Lima beans and pine nuts add bite to the grainy dish, coriander and dill the subtle flavors.

½ medium onion, chopped	⅓ teaspoon ground coriander
1 teaspoon safflower oil	1⅔ cups water
¾ cup white basmati rice	⅓ cup frozen lima beans
1½ tablespoons pine nuts	¼ teaspoon salt
3 tablespoons chopped fresh dill	

1. In a 1½- or 2-quart saucepan sauté the onion in the oil for 2–3 minutes. Add the rice to the onions along with the pine nuts, dill, and coriander, and sauté for 2 minutes.

2. Add the water, lima beans, and salt. Bring to a boil, then cover and reduce to a low simmer. Cook the rice for 15–20 minutes.

Yield: Makes 8 ⅓-cup servings

Each serving has approximately 106 calories, 3.2 g. protein, 3.4 g. total fat (2.6 g. unsaturated fat, 0.5 g. saturated fat), 16.9 g. carbohydrates, 0 mg. cholesterol, 1.6 g. fiber, 72 mg. sodium, 30.2 mg. calcium. Exchanges per serving: ½ fat, 1 starch.

Bulgur Pilaf with Basil and Pine Nuts

An unusual pilaf with a light nutty flavor, the aroma of fresh basil, and the crunch of pine nuts.

2⅔   cups water
1⅓   cups bulgur wheat
 ⅓   cup chopped fresh basil
2½   tablespoons pine nuts
 ⅓   teaspoon freshly ground
      pepper
 ⅓   teaspoon salt

1. Bring the water to a boil and take off heat. Soak the bulgur wheat in the hot water for 45 minutes, or until the water is absorbed.

2. Add the remaining ingredients and mix well.

Yield: Makes 8 ⅓-cup servings

Each serving has approximately 119 calories, 4.1 g. protein, 2.6 g. total fat (2 g. unsaturated fat, 0.5 g. saturated fat), 21.6 g. carbohydrates, 0 mg. cholesterol, 5.1 g. fiber, 89.2 mg. sodium, 9.9 mg. calcium. Exchanges per serving: ½ fat, 1¼ starch.

Wild Rice Frittata

Nutty, chewy, spicy and crunchy.

1¼ cups water	1 teaspoon onion powder
¼ cup brown rice	1 teaspoon garlic powder
¼ cup wild rice	½ teaspoon salt
½ cup fresh cooked corn or frozen kernels, defrosted	¼ teaspoon freshly ground black pepper
½ cup finely chopped carrots	1 egg, lightly beaten
¼ cup finely chopped celery	1 tablespoon corn oil

1. In a 2-quart saucepan, bring 1¼ cups of water to a boil. Add the brown and wild rices, cover, reduce to low heat, and cook for 45 to 50 minutes, or until the water is absorbed.

2. Add the corn, carrots, celery, onion powder, garlic powder, salt, pepper, and egg, and mix well. Pack a ¼-cup measure with the rice mixture, and turn it over onto a sheet of wax paper, then make 7 more rice patties, and set them aside.

3. Preheat oven to 350° F.

4. Heat the oil in a heavy non-stick, 10-inch skillet over medium heat. With a spatula, transfer the patties to the heated skillet, and cook them for 4 minutes. Turn the patties over, placing them as close together as possible, and with the spatula lightly press the tops of the 8 patties together to mold them into one large rice frittata. Cook for 4 more minutes.

5. Lightly coat a baking pan with non-stick cooking spray, or line with foil. Flip the frittata onto the baking pan, and bake for 15 minutes. Cut into 8 pieces and serve.

Yield: Serves 8

Each serving has approximately 68 calories, 3.5 g. protein, 2.7 g. total fat (1.9 g. unsaturated fat, 0.5 g. saturated fat), 17 g. carbohydrates, 26 mg. cholesterol, 0.9 g. fiber, 150 mg. sodium, 13 mg. calcium. Exchanges per serving: ½ fat, ½ starch.

Lemon Couscous

This light, fluffy grain with a hint of lemon is as easy as cooking gets. It's a delectable accompaniment to chicken and lamb.

1⅓ cups water
  2 teaspoons finely grated
    lemon peel
⅔ cup dried couscous

1. In a 1½-quart saucepan bring the water and lemon peel to a boil. Add the couscous, and turn off heat, cover, and let sit for 5 minutes.
2. Fluff with a fork, and serve.

Yield: Makes 8 ⅓-cup servings
Each serving has approximately 40 calories, 1.3 g. protein, 0 g. total fat (0 g. unsaturated fat, 0 g. saturated fat), 8.6 g. carbohydrates, 0 mg. cholesterol, 0.5 g. fiber, 1.65 mg. sodium, 5 mg. calcium.
Exchanges per serving: ½ starch.

Polenta with Pesto

Polenta, a staple in Italy, is cooked cornmeal. Pesto adds the strong flavor of basil.

  3 cups water
1¼ cups yellow cornmeal
  3 ounces grated Parmesan
    cheese
  1 Recipe Pesto Genovese
    (page 132)

1. In a heavy 2-quart saucepan bring the water to a boil. Slowly sprinkle the cornmeal into the water, stirring constantly to avoid lumps. As soon as the mixture gets very thick, reduce the heat to low. When it starts to pull away from the sides of the pan, stir in the Parmesan cheese and cook for 30 seconds more.
2. Pour the polenta into an 8 × 8-inch baking pan with 2-inch-high sides, and let cool.
3. Make the pesto Genovese.

4. Spread the pesto evenly over the cornmeal. Cut the cornmeal into 16 squares and serve.

Yield: Makes 16 2-inch squares

Each square has approximately 91 calories, 4 g. protein, 4.7 g. total fat (2.8 g. unsaturated fat, 1.5 g. saturated fat), 9.3 g. carbohydrates, 4.8 mg. cholesterol, 1.6 g. fiber, 209 mg. sodium, 154 mg. calcium. Exchanges per serving: ⅕ meat, 1 starch.

Speckled Kasha

A light, fluffy, nutty-tasting grain, also called buckwheat, with colorful bites of several vegetables.

1 garlic clove, finely chopped	1½ cups Basic Chicken Stock
½ small onion, finely chopped	(page 86)
1 medium carrot, peeled and	¾ cup whole groat kasha
finely chopped	(buckwheat)
1 celery stalk, finely chopped	⅓ teaspoon salt
⅓ cup fresh or frozen and	½ teaspoon black pepper
defrosted lima beans	2 teaspoons chopped fresh
	thyme

1. In a 2-quart saucepan sauté the garlic, onion, carrot, celery, and lima beans for 2 minutes with 1 tablespoon of the chicken stock.
2. Rinse the kasha in a fine mesh colander under cold water for 30 seconds. Add to the vegetables in the saucepan, then stir in the stock, salt, pepper, and thyme. Bring to a boil, reduce heat to low, and cook, covered, for 10 minutes.

Yield: Makes 8 ½-cup servings

Each serving has approximately 72 calories, 3 g. protein, 0.5 g. total fat (0.3 g. unsaturated fat, 0.1 g. saturated fat), 16 g. carbohydrates, 0 mg. cholesterol, 3 g. fiber, 97 mg. sodium, 32 mg. calcium. Exchanges per serving: ⅔ starch, 1 vegetable.

Chinese Noodles with Asparagus

Crunchy vegetables in a spicy piquant sauce.

4 ounces plain uncooked
 Chinese noodles
2 carrots
1 pound asparagus
1 tablespoon sesame tahini
1 tablespoon toasted sesame oil
2 tablespoons low-sodium soy
 sauce

1 tablespoon dry sherry
1 tablespoon rice vinegar
½ teaspoon crushed red pepper
 flakes
2 tablespoons chopped fresh
 basil

1. Cook the Chinese noodles in 2 quarts of boiling water for 3 minutes. Drain through a colander, and place the noodles in a large bowl.

2. Peel the carrots, trim roots, and cut into julienne strips. Trim the ends of the asparagus, and cut the stalks into 1-inch diagonals.

3. Steam the carrots and asparagus until fork-tender, or microwave, covered, on high heat for 3 minutes. Add the vegetables to the noodles.

4. Combine the remaining ingredients until smooth and creamy, pour over the noodles and vegetables, and toss to coat evenly.

Yield: Makes 4 1-cup servings

Each serving has approximately 217 calories, 8.8 g. protein, 7.1 g. total fat (5.3 g. unsaturated fat, 1.1 g. saturated fat), 30.8 g. carbohydrates, 27.5 mg. cholesterol, 5.2 g. fiber, 319 mg. sodium, 81.9 mg. calcium. Exchanges per serving: 1 fat, ¼ meat, 1½ starch, 1 vegetable.

Pasta Tutti

Slightly spicy with a light fresh anise flavor. We call it Pasta Tutti because it has practically everything but the kitchen sink.

1 medium eggplant	1 tablespoon capers
3 garlic cloves, finely chopped	⅓ teaspoon salt
½ cup chopped onions	¼ cup finely chopped fresh basil
½ cup finely chopped fennel stems	¼ teaspoon crushed red pepper or freshly ground pepper to taste
½ teaspoon corn oil	
3 cups canned, peeled tomatoes, including juice, diced	6 ounces rigatoni, pasta shells, tubes, or elbow pasta
	4 teaspoons Parmesan cheese

1. Pierce the eggplant with a fork two or three times.
2. To bake in oven, preheat oven to 425° F. Place the eggplant on a baking sheet and bake for 40 minutes.

   To microwave, place the eggplant in a microwave-safe dish and cook on high, uncovered, for 8 minutes.
3. After the eggplant has cooked, cut it in half to let the steam escape, and let it cool for 10 minutes. Then remove the skin and stem, lightly chop the pulp, and set it aside.
4. In a heavy 2-quart sauce pan sauté the garlic, onions, and fennel in the corn oil for 3 minutes. Add the eggplant, tomatoes, capers, salt, basil, and pepper, and cook over low heat for 10 minutes.
5. Cook the pasta according to package instructions, but not using any salt or oil. Drain well.
6. Add the pasta to the sauce and toss gently. Transfer to a warmed serving platter and sprinkle the Parmesan cheese on top.

Yield: Serves 4

Each serving has approximately 245 calories, 10 g. protein, 2.3 g. total fat (1.3 g. unsaturated fat, 0.6 g. saturated fat), 49 g. carbohydrates, 1.3 mg. cholesterol, 7.7 g. fiber, 570 mg. sodium, 173 mg. calcium. Exchanges per serving: ½ fat, 2 starch, 2½ vegetable.

Angel Hair with Scallops and Crabmeat

Tender pasta and crisp vegetables in a fresh herbed tomato sauce.

3 or 4	large, ripe, fresh tomatoes (for 4 cups tomato puree)	½	tablespoon olive oil
2	garlic cloves, finely chopped	½	cup chopped fresh basil or 2 teaspoons dried
½	teaspoon crushed red pepper	½	tablespoon chopped fresh thyme or 1 teaspoon dried
1	leek, trimmed and thinly sliced (3 ounces trimmed)	¼	teaspoon salt
		4	ounces bay scallops
		2	ounces crabmeat, shredded
1	small red bell pepper, cut into very fine strips	12	ounces dried angel hair

1. Seed and peel the tomatoes, then puree in a blender until smooth. Set aside.

2. In a 2-quart saucepan sauté the garlic, crushed red pepper, leek, and bell pepper strips in the oil for 2 minutes. Add the tomato puree, basil, thyme, and salt, and cook for 10 minutes, uncovered, over low heat, stirring frequently.

3. Add the scallops and crabmeat, and continue cooking for 5 minutes.

4. Meanwhile, cook the pasta according to package directions, but not using any salt or oil. Drain and transfer to a warm platter, pour the sauce over the pasta, and serve.

Yield: Serves 8

Each serving has approximately 251 calories, 12.2 g. protein, 3 g. total fat (1.9 g. unsaturated fat, 0.6 g. saturated fat), 45.8 g. carbohydrates, 12 mg. cholesterol, 6.3 g. fiber, 151 mg. sodium, 67 mg. calcium. Exchanges per serving: ¾ meat, 2 starch, 2 vegetable.

Fettuccine with Mushroom Stroganoff

We used fettuccine, but you can choose your favorite pasta for this rich and creamy sauce.

2 garlic cloves, finely chopped	½ cup unsalted, fat-free chicken stock
½ small onion, finely chopped	
2 tablespoons dry sherry	¼ cup reduced-fat sour cream
3½ ounces fresh shiitake mushrooms, trimmed of stems and sliced	¼ cup plain non-fat yogurt
	½ teaspoon salt
	½ teaspoon freshly ground black pepper
1 pound regular button mushrooms, sliced	1½ tablespoons chopped fresh dill
1 tablespoon margarine	
1 tablespoon unbleached flour	4 ounces fettuccine

1. In a non-stick 10-inch sauté pan cook the garlic and onion with the sherry for 2 minutes. Add the sliced shiitake and button mushrooms, and cook for 4 minutes over medium heat, until the mushrooms are soft. Transfer the entire mixture to a bowl and set aside.

2. Using the same pan, melt the margarine. Sprinkle the flour on top, stirring to make a smooth roux, and cook for 1 minute.

3. Slowly add the chicken stock, stirring constantly to break up any lumps. The sauce should start to thicken. After all the chicken stock is added and the sauce has some body, stir in the mushroom mixture, and heat for 3 minutes.

4. Reduce the sauce to low, then stir a tablespoon of hot sauce into the sour cream to prevent curdling. Add all the sour cream and yogurt to the mushroom mixture, and stir until creamy. Add the salt, pepper, and dill, and cook over low heat until the sauce is hot.

5. Meanwhile, prepare the fettuccine according to package instructions, but not using any salt or oil, then drain, and serve on a warm platter topped with the hot sauce.

Yield: Serves 4

Each serving has approximately 240 calories, 9 g. protein, 6.9 g. total fat (4.1 g. unsaturated fat, 2 g. saturated fat), 35 g. carbohydrates, 0.3 mg. cholesterol, 5.4 g. fiber, 342 mg. sodium, 67 mg. calcium. Exchanges per serving: 1 fat, ¼ milk, 1⅔ starch, 2 vegetable.

Vegetable Lasagna

Three chewy vegetables combined with tender pasta, slightly salty cheese, and tangy tomato sauce.

9 lasagna noodles, each 2 × 11 inches (7 ounces)
1 medium eggplant
10 ounces fresh spinach or frozen spinach, defrosted
1 pound mushrooms, sliced
4 small garlic cloves
¼ cup fresh basil leaves, packed

½ cup part-skim ricotta cheese
2 cups low-fat (1%) cottage cheese
2 cups Italian Spaghetti Sauce with Fresh Herbs (page 136)
3 ounces part-skim mozzarella cheese, grated
½ cup Parmesan cheese, grated (2 ounces)

1. Preheat oven to 400° F.

2. In a large pot, boil the lasagna noodles according to package instructions, but not using any salt or oil.

3. Prick the eggplant with a knife a few times, and bake for 40 minutes or microwave for 10 minutes on high.

4. Meanwhile, in a 10-inch fry pan sauté the spinach until wilted, about 5 minutes. Drain in a colander to remove excess moisture. Do the same for the mushrooms.

5. In a food processor chop the garlic and basil until fine. Add the ricotta cheese and cottage cheese, and puree for 30 seconds.

6. When the eggplant has cooked, cut it in half to let the steam escape, and let it cool for 10 minutes. Scrape the eggplant meat into a bowl and set aside. Reduce oven heat to 375° F.

7. To assemble the dish, spoon 1 cup of the spaghetti sauce on the bottom of the pan, then lay 3 lasagna noodles lengthwise in a 9 × 11 × 2-inch pan. Carefully spread the ricotta–cottage cheese mixture evenly over the noodles. Cover the cheese with 3 more noodles. Spread the spinach, then the mushrooms, and finally the eggplant over the noodles, and cover the vegetables with the mozzarella and Parmesan cheeses. Over that place a final layer of noodles, then the remaining cup of spaghetti sauce.

8. Cover with foil and bake for 30 minutes. Remove the foil, and bake for 10 more minutes. Remove the lasagna from the oven and let it rest for 10 minutes before serving.

Yield: Serves 8

Each serving has approximately 249 calories, 19 g. protein, 5.5 g. total fat (2.3 g. unsaturated fat, 2.1 g. saturated fat), 33 g. carbohydrates, 13 mg. cholesterol, 7.7 g. fiber, 400 mg. sodium, 246 mg. calcium. Exchanges per serving: 1½ meat, 1¼ starch, 2½ vegetable.

Lasagna Roll-ups

Lasagna in a different form—individual rolls with low-fat cheese filling and spaghetti sauce.

3½ quarts water	¼ teaspoon freshly ground
8 lasagna noodles, each 2 × 11 inches	black pepper
2 cups part-skim ricotta cheese	1½ cups Italian Spaghetti Sauce with Fresh Herbs (page 136)
2 garlic cloves, finely chopped	¼ cup coarsely grated Parmesan cheese (1 ounce)
2 tablespoons chopped fresh basil or 2 teaspoons dried	

1. Preheat oven to 350° F.
2. In a large pot boil the noodles according to package instructions, but not using any salt or oil. Carefully remove them from the pot and drain on paper towels.
3. In a large bowl combine the ricotta cheese, garlic, basil, and pepper.
4. Pour half the spaghetti sauce on the bottom of a 10-inch bake-and-serve dish with 3-inch sides.
5. Lay one cooked noodle on a board, and 1 inch in from one end spoon ¼ cup of the ricotta mixture. Roll the noodle over the cheese, and roll it the length of the noodle to form an open-sided roulade. Lay it seam side down over the sauce in the pan. Repeat for the other noodles.
6. Pour the remaining sauce over the roll-ups, then sprinkle them with the Parmesan cheese. Cover and bake for 20 minutes.

Yield: Makes 8 roll-ups

Each roll-up has approximately 183 calories, 10.3 g. protein, 7.3 g. total fat (3.4 g. unsaturated fat, 3.4 g. saturated fat), 19.5 g. carbohydrates, 34.5 mg. cholesterol, 1.7 g. fiber, 247 mg. sodium, 192 mg. calcium.
Exchanges per serving: 1½ meat, 1 starch, 1 vegetable.

Pasta Fagioli

Macaroni bathed in a tomato sauce packed with basil, licorice-flavored fennel, juicy zucchini, and chewy chick-peas.

3 ounces macaroni	5 fresh medium-size plum tomatoes, quartered
2 teaspoons olive oil	
2 garlic cloves, finely chopped	1 can (19-ounce) cooked chick-peas, drained
1½ cups sliced fennel, ¼ inch thick	1 cup lightly chopped fresh basil
1½ cups sliced zucchini, ⅓ inch thick	½ teaspoon freshly ground pepper

1. Cook the macaroni according to package directions, but without any salt or oil. Drain in a colander.

2. Meanwhile, in a heavy 2-quart saucepan heat the oil, and sauté the garlic, fennel, and zucchini for 2 minutes. Add the plum tomatoes, and cook for 2 minutes. Stir in the chick-peas, basil, pepper, and cooked pasta, and cook for 5 minutes over low heat.

Yield: Serves 4

Each serving has approximately 274 calories, 12.3 g. protein, 5.5 g. total fat (4 g. unsaturated fat, 0.8 g. saturated fat), 46 g. carbohydrates, 0 mg. cholesterol, 10 g. fiber, 68 mg. sodium, 90 mg. calcium. Exchanges per serving: ½ fat, 2½ starch, 1½ vegetable.

Penne with Basil and Sweet Peppers

Crisp bell pepper strips, juicy fresh tomatoes, and basil leaves to dress a pasta of your choice. Serve it lukewarm, or as a cool salad.

6 ounces penne, or any other pasta	¼ pound fresh plum tomatoes (about 3), cut into eighths
1 medium red bell pepper, cut in half, then into strips	2 garlic cloves, finely chopped
1 medium yellow bell pepper, cut in half, then into strips	1½ tablespoons olive oil
	½ teaspoon freshly ground pepper
1 bunch fresh basil leaves (¾ cup packed)	½ teaspoon salt

1. Cook the pasta according to package directions, omitting any oil and salt. Drain through a colander.

2. In a large bowl combine the remaining ingredients, and add the cooked pasta. Toss to mix well. Serve at once, or let cool.

Yield: Serves 4

Each serving has approximately 235 calories, 7 g. protein, 7 g. total fat (5.3 g. unsaturated fat, 1.2 g. saturated fat), 36.8 g. carbohydrates, 0 mg. cholesterol, 4.8 g. fiber, 288 mg. sodium, 30.8 mg. calcium. Exchanges per serving: 1 fat, 2 starch, 1 vegetable.

Linguine and Lobster

Bits of sweet lobster in a creamy sauce.

1 pound live lobster (¼ pound lobster meat)	1¼ cups skim milk
6 ounces linguini	½ cup grated Parmesan cheese
1 large shallot, finely chopped	¼ teaspoon salt
2 garlic cloves, finely chopped	1 teaspoon fresh crushed rosemary, or ¾ teaspoon dried
1 tablespoon white wine	⅓ teaspoon freshly ground pepper
1 tablespoon margarine	
1 tablespoon flour	

1. In a large pot cook the lobster in 2 quarts of boiling water for 5 minutes. Remove the lobster from the pot, and let it cool. Crack the shells to remove the lobster meat, and cut it into bite-sized pieces.

2. In the large pot cook the linguini according to package instructions, without extra oil or salt.

3. Meanwhile, in a heavy 10-inch sauté pan cook the shallot and garlic in white wine for 1 minute, until the wine evaporates. Add the margarine, and let it melt over medium heat. Stir in the flour, and cook for only 1 minute, stirring constantly. Still stirring, slowly add the milk, then the cheese, salt, rosemary, and pepper. Cook over very low heat until the sauce thickens, about 2 minutes. Add the lobster meat and cook for 2 more minutes.

4. Drain the pasta in a colander, transfer it to a warm serving platter, and pour the lobster sauce over.

Yield: Serves 4

Each serving has approximately 258 calories, 14 g. protein, 5.1 g. total fat (3.5 g. unsaturated fat, 1.2 g. saturated fat), 37 g. carbohydrates, 22 mg. cholesterol, 3 g. fiber, 282 mg. sodium, 142 mg. calcium. Exchanges per serving: ½ fat, 1½ meat, ⅓ milk, 1½ starch.

Linguine with Tomato Clam Sauce

Pasta dressed with basil, tomatoes and their juices, flecks of parsley, and bites of clam.

12 ounces linguini	¼ cup chopped fresh basil or
3 garlic cloves, finely chopped	2 teaspoons dried basil (omit
1 tablespoon olive oil	if using canned tomatoes that
1 can (28-ounce) crushed	include basil)
tomatoes or 3½ cups coarsely	2 cans (6½ ounces each) minced
chopped and seeded fresh	clams, including juice
plum tomatoes	½ teaspoon freshly ground black
	pepper
	¼ cup chopped fresh parsley

1. Cook the pasta according to package instructions, but without any salt or oil. Drain in a colander.

2. Meanwhile, in a 2½-quart saucepan, sauté the garlic in oil for 30 seconds. Add the tomatoes, basil, and clams (including clam juice), pepper, and parsley. Simmer on low while the pasta cooks. The sauce will reduce slightly in volume.

3. Serve the sauce over the pasta.

Yield: Serves 4

Each serving has approximately 255 calories, 18.4 g. protein, 5.9 g. total fat (4.1 g. unsaturated fat, 0.9 g. saturated fat), 32.5 g. carbohydrates, 59.3 mg. cholesterol, 4.3 g. fiber, 492 mg. sodium, 127 mg. calcium.

Exchanges per serving: ½ fat, 1½ meat, 1½ starch, 1 vegetable.

Spicy Italian "Meatballs" with Spaghetti

Spicy turkey balls in Italian Spaghetti Sauce with Fresh Herbs (page 136) over spaghetti.

½	pound ground turkey	¼	teaspoon crushed red pepper flakes
⅛	teaspoon salt		
¼	teaspoon white pepper	2	tablespoons tomato sauce
1	teaspoon ground coriander	1½	tablespoons fine dry bread crumbs
¼	teaspoon garlic powder		
½	teaspoon oregano	4	cups Italian Spaghetti Sauce with Fresh Herbs (page 136)
¾	teaspoon ground fennel		
		10	ounces spaghetti

1. In a large bowl combine the ground turkey, salt, white pepper, coriander, garlic powder, oregano, fennel, red pepper flakes, tomato sauce, and bread crumbs. Roll into 16 small meatballs.

2. Lightly coat a 10-inch non-stick fry pan with non-stick cooking spray, and heat it over medium heat. Add half the meatballs, cook for 1 minute, turn them over, and cook for 1 more minute. Repeat for all raw sections, cooking for 1 minute each time until there are no raw spots, then cook for 1 more minute. Transfer to a warm serving dish and repeat with the remaining meatballs.

Or in a microwave-safe dish cook the meatballs on high for 3 minutes, rotating the dish after 1½ minutes.

3. In a saucepan combine the spaghetti sauce with the meatballs, and cook over medium heat for 5 minutes.

4. Meanwhile, cook the pasta according to package directions, but without extra oil or salt.

5. Drain the pasta in a colander, transfer to a warm serving platter, pour over the sauce and meatballs, and serve.

Yield: Serves 8

Each serving has approximately 270 calories, 13.2 g. protein, 8.3 g. total fat (6 g. unsaturated fat, 1.7 g. saturated fat), 38 g. carbohydrates, 24 mg. cholesterol, 3.9 g. fiber, 560 mg. sodium, 53 mg. calcium. Exchanges per serving: 1 fat, 1 meat, 1¾ starch, 1 vegetable.

Breads, Biscuits, and Such

Cranberry Nut Bread
Pumpkin Bread
Whole Wheat Blueberry
   Muffins
Banana Walnut Muffins
Applesauce Walnut Bran
   Muffins
Sweet Potato Biscuits
Poppy Seed Biscuits
Cinnamon Buns
Rye Dinner Rolls
Herbed Whole Wheat Bread
   Sticks

Jalapeño Corn Biscuits
Kasha Knishes
Bagel Chips
Homemade Tortilla Chips
Homemade Flour Tortillas
   with Scallions
Corn Pancakes
Blintzes
Blueberry Oatmeal Pancakes
Perfect Crepes

Cranberry Nut Bread

Tart and nutty with a light, fluffy texture.

1 tablespoon oil	1 teaspoon baking powder
⅓ cup brown sugar	½ teaspoon baking soda
1½ cups buttermilk	¼ teaspoon salt
1 egg, lightly beaten	2 tablespoons chopped walnuts
1 cup whole wheat flour	1 cup fresh cranberries, finely
1 cup unbleached flour	chopped

1. Preheat oven to 425° F. Lightly coat a 5×9-inch loaf pan with non-stick cooking spray.

2. In a large bowl mix the oil and sugar. Add the buttermilk and beaten egg, stirring until smooth.

3. In another bowl combine the remaining ingredients, and add to the liquid mixture, stirring just until the batter is moistened. Don't overmix it.

4. Pour the batter evenly into the prepared pan, and bake for 30 minutes, or until golden brown.

Yield: Makes 18 ½-inch slices

Each serving has approximately 89 calories, 2.8 g. protein, 1.8 g. total fat (1.4 g. unsaturated fat, 0.3 g. saturated fat), 16 g. carbohydrates, 1 mg. cholesterol, 1.3 g. fiber, 85 mg. sodium, 45 mg. calcium.
Exchanges per serving: ⅓ fat, 1 starch.

Pumpkin Bread

Sweet, spicy, and chewy bread dotted with raisins.

3 tablespoons oil	¾ cup whole wheat flour
2 tablespoons brown sugar	1 cup unbleached white flour
1 egg	1 teaspoon baking powder
1 cup canned pumpkin puree	1 teaspoon baking soda
⅓ cup molasses	¼ teaspoon allspice
½ cup plus 1 tablespoon butter-milk	1 teaspoon cinnamon
	¼ cup raisins

1. Preheat oven to 400° F. Lightly coat a 5×9-inch loaf pan with non-stick cooking spray.

2. In a large bowl, beat the oil, sugar, and egg together. Add the pumpkin puree, molasses, and buttermilk, and mix well.

3. In another bowl combine the whole wheat flour, white flour, baking powder, baking soda, allspice, cinnamon, and raisins together well. Add them to the sugar-egg mixture, and stir to combine.

4. Pour the batter into the prepared pan, and bake for 45 minutes.

Yield: Makes 18 ½-inch slices

Each slice has approximately 86 calories, 2.2 g. protein, 2.8 g. total fat (2.2 g. unsaturated fat, 0.4 g. saturated fat), 13.6 g. carbohydrates, 11.7 mg. cholesterol, 1.2 g. fiber, 71 mg. sodium, 32 mg. calcium. Exchanges per serving: ½ fat, ¾ starch.

Whole Wheat Blueberry Muffins

Nice crumb, extra texture from the whole wheat flour, and a slight burst of fruity blueberries in these mini-muffins.

1 cup less 1 tablespoon whole wheat flour	⅓ cup brown sugar
1 cup less 1 tablespoon unbleached flour	1 egg
2 teaspoons baking powder	1 cup skim milk
½ teaspoon salt	1 cup fresh blueberries, or unsweetened frozen blue-
2 tablespoons corn oil	berries, defrosted

1. Preheat oven to 400° F. Lightly coat with non-stick cooking spray enough muffin tins with 1⅝-inch cups to make 24 muffins.

2. In a medium-sized mixing bowl, combine the whole wheat and unbleached flours with the baking powder and salt.

3. In another bowl, combine the oil, sugar, egg, and skim milk. Add these liquid ingredients to the dry ingredients, stirring until moistened. Add the blueberries to the batter and stir lightly to combine.

4. Spoon the batter into the prepared muffin tins, and bake for 16–18 minutes, or until muffins are lightly brown and firm.

Yield: Makes 24 1⅝-inch muffins

Each muffin has approximately 66 calories, 1.8 g. protein, 1.5 g. total fat (0.6 g. unsaturated fat, 0.3 g. saturated fat), 11.7 g. carbohydrates, 8.8 mg. cholesterol, 0.9 g. fiber, 82 mg. sodium, 24.5 mg. calcium. Exchanges per serving: ¼ fat, ⅔ starch.

Banana Walnut Muffins

Chewy, rich, banana flavor with the added crunch of nuts.

½ cup unbleached flour
1 cup whole wheat flour
¼ cup unprocessed oat bran
1 teaspoon baking powder
½ teaspoon baking soda
1 teaspoon cinnamon
¼ teaspoon salt
2 tablespoons finely chopped walnuts

1 tablespoon corn oil
¼ cup brown sugar
2 egg whites
1 cup mashed ripe banana (1½ large bananas)
1 cup plus 1 tablespoon non-fat buttermilk

1. Preheat oven to 425° F. Lightly coat the muffin tin with non-stick cooking spray.
2. In a large bowl combine the unbleached and whole wheat flours, oat bran, baking powder, baking soda, cinnamon, salt, and walnuts.
3. In a separate bowl mix the oil, sugar, egg whites, and banana together with an electric mixer. Stir in the buttermilk.
4. Add the banana mixture to the dry ingredients, stirring only until the batter is moist. Spoon the batter into the prepared muffin tin and bake for 18–20 minutes, or until a cake tester comes out dry.

Yield: Makes 12 2½-inch muffins

Each muffin has approximately 119 calories, 3.9 g. protein, 2.4 g. total fat (2 g. unsaturated fat, 0.3 g. saturated fat), 23 g. carbohydrates, 0.4 mg. cholesterol, 2.2 g. fiber, 126 mg. sodium, 57 mg. calcium. Exchanges per serving: ½ fat, ¼ fruit, 1 starch.

Applesauce Walnut Bran Muffins

Chewy muffins with lots of texture. Very filling!

1 tablespoon corn oil	1 teaspoon baking powder
½ cup brown sugar	1 teaspoon baking soda
2 egg whites	½ teaspoon salt
⅔ cup unsweetened applesauce	2 teaspoons cinnamon
⅔ cup skim milk	¾ cup old fashioned rolled oats
¾ cup unbleached flour	¼ cup chopped walnuts
¾ cup wheat bran	

1. Preheat oven to 350° F. Lightly coat with non-stick cooking spray a muffin tin with 12 2½-inch cups.

2. Cream the oil and sugar together until smooth. Add the egg whites, applesauce, and skim milk, and mix well.

3. In a large bowl, combine the flour, wheat bran, baking powder, baking soda, salt, cinnamon, oats, and walnuts.

4. Pour the creamed mixture into the dry ingredients, and stir until smooth. Spoon into the prepared muffin tin, and bake for 22–25 minutes, or until the muffins are slightly firm to the touch.

Yield: Makes 12 2½-inch muffins

Each muffin has approximately 125 calories, 3.3 g. protein, 3.2 g. total fat (2.7 g. unsaturated fat, 0.3 g. saturated fat), 22.2 g. carbohydrates, 0.2 mg. cholesterol, 2.2 g. fiber, 202 mg. sodium, 54.7 mg. calcium. Exchanges per serving: ¼ fat, 1¼ starch.

Sweet Potato Biscuits

Tender biscuits, with the warm flavor of cinnamon and slight sweetness of the potato.

½ pound sweet potato	¼ teaspoon salt
¼ teaspoon cinnamon	1½ tablespoons chilled marga-
¼ teaspoon allspice	rine, cut into small chunks
1¼ cups sifted, unbleached flour	¼ cup skim milk
2 teaspoons baking powder	

1. Preheat oven to 425° F. Lightly coat a cookie sheet with non-stick cooking spray.

2. Prick the sweet potato with a fork and bake in the oven for 1 hour, or cook in microwave on high for 8 minutes.

3. Combine the cinnamon, allspice, flour, baking powder, and salt in a food processor. Add the margarine, and pulse 6 or 7 times, until slightly crumbly.

Or combine these dry ingredients in a bowl, and cut in the chilled margarine with a pastry cutter or two forks.

4. Add ¾ cup of the baked sweet potato meat, and mix until crumbly.

5. Add the milk a tablespoon at a time until a soft, kneadable dough is formed. You may not need all the milk.

6. Place the dough on a lightly floured board, and knead it for 30 seconds. Roll it out to ½-inch thickness, and cut 12 rounds, using a 1½-inch biscuit cutter. You will have to reshape and reroll the dough several times to utilize all the dough for the biscuits.

7. Lay the rounds of dough on the prepared pan, and bake for 10–12 minutes, or until the tops are lightly browned.

Yield: Makes 12 biscuits

Each biscuit has approximately 74 calories, 1.6 g. protein, 1.6 g. total fat (1.2 g. unsaturated fat, 0.3 g. saturated fat), 13 g. carbohydrates, 0.1 mg. cholesterol, 0.8 g. fiber, 114 mg. sodium, 43.4 mg. calcium. Exchanges per serving: 1 starch.

Poppy Seed Biscuits

Very light, slightly sweet biscuits dotted with poppy seeds.

1 cup unbleached flour	1 tablespoon poppy seeds
¼ cup whole wheat flour	1½ tablespoons chilled marga-
2 teaspoons baking powder	rine, cut into small pieces
¼ teaspoon salt	½ cup skim milk
2 tablespoons sugar	

1. Preheat oven to 425° F. Lightly coat a cookie pan with non-stick cooking spray.
2. In a bowl or food processor, combine the flours, baking powder, salt, sugar, and poppy seeds.
3. Cut the margarine into the flour until crumbly, using a fork or the metal chopping blade of the food processor.
4. Add the skim milk, stirring until the batter is moist, firm, and pulls away from the sides of the bowl.
5. Transfer the dough to a lightly floured board. Knead it for 1 minute. Roll the dough out to a ½-inch thickness with a rolling pin. Using a 1-inch biscuit cutter, cut out 14 biscuits. You will have to reshape and reroll the dough at least once to form all the biscuits. Lay the biscuits on the prepared cookie sheet, and bake for 8–10 minutes, until lightly browned.

Yield: Makes 14 1-inch biscuits

Each biscuit has approximately 48 calories, 1.3 g. protein, 1.2 g. total fat (0.9 g. unsaturated fat, 0.2 g. saturated fat), 7.8 g. carbohydrates, 0.1 mg. cholesterol, 0.5 g. fiber, 91 mg. sodium, 19.3 mg. calcium. Exchanges per serving: ⅔ starch.

Cinnamon Buns

Light yeasty buns with a spicy flavor.

1 cup warm water	½ teaspoon salt
1 package active dry yeast	2½ cups unbleached flour
1 tablespoon granulated sugar	1 tablespoon cinnamon
½ cup warm skim milk	3 tablespoons brown sugar
¾ cup whole wheat flour	2 tablespoons stick margarine

1. Pour the warm water into a medium-sized mixing bowl. Sprinkle the yeast and the granulated sugar on top. Cover the bowl with a towel, and let it sit for 5 minutes in a draft-free area.

2. Add the warm milk and the whole wheat flour, and stir to moisten. Cover with the towel, and let it sit for 10 minutes in a draft-free space.

3. Add the salt and 1 cup of the unbleached flour, ¼ cup at a time, and stir until the dough starts to pull away from the sides of the bowl.

4. At this point, add ½ cup of the remaining flour to a pastry board or clean counter top, and transfer the dough to the floured surface. Lightly oil your hands to prevent sticking while you knead the dough. Push the dough away from you with the palms of your hands, then pull it back with your fingertips. As you knead, the dough will absorb the flour on the board, and you may need to add about 1 more tablespoon. (The amount of flour depends on the moisture content of the flour and humidity in the air.) Knead the dough for 5 minutes, until it is light and springy. Transfer the dough to a clean, lightly oiled bowl. Cover with a towel, and let sit in a draft-free space for 1 hour, or until the dough doubles in bulk.

5. When the dough has risen, punch it down with your fist. Dust 1 tablespoon of the remaining flour on the board, and knead the dough again for 1 minute. Divide dough into 2 equal pieces, and set one aside.

6. Dust the board with 1 more tablespoon of the flour, and roll one of the pieces of dough to about 8 × 10 inches and about ¼ inch thick, with the wider side facing you. Sprinkle ½ tablespoon of the cinnamon over it, then sprinkle 1½ tablespoons of the brown sugar over the cinnamon, and spread to coat evenly. Cut half the margarine into 32 tiny bits and dot them over the dough.

7. Cut the dough in half the long way, into two 4×10-inch rectangles. Roll each one up like a jelly-roll, starting at the bottom. You will now have two 10-inch logs about 2 inches in diameter. Cut each log into 5 pieces.

8. Lightly coat two large baking pans, each about 18 × 13 inches, with non-stick cooking spray. Lay the cinnamon rolls on the pans, flat side down, about 2 inches apart.

9. Repeat this procedure with the remaining dough, and let all the cinnamon buns rise for 30 minutes.

10. Preheat the oven to 375° F. Bake the buns for 15 minutes.

Yield: Makes 20 2-inch rolls

Each bun has approximately 96 calories, 2.6 g. protein, 1.4 g. total fat (1 g. unsaturated fat, 0.3 g. saturated fat), 18.4 g. carbohydrates, 0.1 mg. cholesterol, 1.2 g. fiber, 71.5 mg. sodium, 19 mg. calcium. Exchanges per serving: 1 starch.

Rye Dinner Rolls

Grainy, chewy rolls with lots of texture.

⅓ cup skim milk	¼ teaspoon salt
½ cup water	¾ cup rye flour
2 teaspoons sugar	1 tablespoon caraway seeds
1 tablespoon corn oil	3 tablespoons unbleached flour
1 envelope active dry yeast	1 teaspoon corn oil
¾ cup whole wheat flour	

1. Warm the milk and water, then pour them in a bowl and stir in the sugar and oil. Sprinkle the yeast on top, then stir for 10 seconds. Cover the bowl with a towel, and let it sit for 5 minutes in a draft-free area.

2. Add the whole wheat flour, and stir for 10 seconds to moisten the flour. Let it sit for 10 minutes, covered, in a draft-free area.

3. Stir in the salt, rye flour, and caraway seeds a little at a time. The dough should begin to pull away from the sides of the bowl.

4. Dust a cutting board or counter top with about 1 tablespoon of the unbleached flour. Lightly oil your hands with ½ teaspoon of the corn oil. Transfer the dough to the floured board, and knead it by pushing the dough away lightly with the heels of your hands, then pulling it back with your fingers. Knead the dough for 5 minutes, adding up to another tablespoon of the flour to the board if necessary, a little at a time. It is important not to add too much flour; the dough can be slightly sticky.

5. Put the dough in a clean bowl that has been lightly oiled. Cover with a towel, and let it rise in a warm place for 45 minutes, or until the dough doubles in bulk.

6. Preheat oven to 375° F. Lightly coat a cookie sheet with non-stick cooking spray.

7. Lightly oil your hands with the remaining ½ teaspoon of corn oil, and dust the cutting board or counter top with the remaining

1 tablespoon of unbleached flour. Punch the dough down in the bowl, then knead it on the lightly floured board or counter for 1 minute.

8. Divide the dough into 12 pieces. Roll each piece into a 3-inch strip, and twist it like a pretzel. Place the formed dough on the prepared cooking sheet and bake for 20 minutes, until lightly browned. Store the baked rolls in an airtight plastic bag in the refrigerator or freezer to preserve freshness.

Yield: Makes 12 rolls

Each roll has approximately 75 calories, 2.6 g. protein, 1.5 g. total fat (1.2 g. unsaturated fat, 0.2 g. saturated fat), 13.6 g. carbohydrates, 0.1 mg. cholesterol, 2.3 g. fiber, 49 mg. sodium, 18 mg. calcium. Exchanges per serving: 1 starch.

Herbed Whole Wheat Bread Sticks

A chewy bread stick with a grainy texture from the whole wheat flour, speckled with fresh herbs and spices. Try them with Creamy Herb Dip (page 125).

½ cup warm water	¾ teaspoon fresh dill or ½ teaspoon dried
½ package active dry yeast (½ tablespoon)	¾ teaspoon fresh thyme or ½ teaspoon dried
½ tablespoon sugar	¾ teaspoon fresh rosemary, lightly chopped, or ½ teaspoon dried
¼ cup skim milk, warm or room temperature	
¼ teaspoon salt	
1¼ cup unbleached flour	¾ teaspoon caraway seeds
6 tablespoons whole wheat flour	1 egg white, lightly beaten
¾ teaspoon fresh chives or ½ teaspoon dried	2 teaspoons onion powder

1. Pour the warm water in a medium-sized bowl. Sprinkle the yeast and sugar on top. Cover the bowl with a towel and let it sit in a warm draft-free area for 5 minutes.

2. Stir in the warm skim milk, salt, and ⅞ cup of the unbleached flour and all of the whole wheat flour, ¼ cup at a time. The dough should start to pull away from the sides of the bowl.

3. Lightly oil your hands.

4. Sprinkle ¼ cup of the remaining flour on a pastry board or counter, and knead the dough for 5 minutes. Transfer the dough to a clean, lightly oiled bowl, cover, and let rise in a warm place for 45 minutes, or until doubled in size.

5. Meanwhile, combine the chives, dill, thyme, rosemary, and caraway seeds in a bowl, and set aside.

6. Lightly coat a large cookie sheet with non-stick cooking spray.

7. Punch the dough down with your fist. Sprinkle 1 tablespoon of flour on the pastry board, and knead the dough for 1 minute.

8. Roll the dough into a rectangle 8 × 10 inches. Sprinkle the herbs over the dough. Roll up the dough like a jelly roll, then knead the entire mixture to distribute the herbs throughout the dough.

9. Break the dough into 4 equal pieces, then cut each of them into 5 individual pieces. Roll the small pieces between your hands to form "ropes" about 5 inches long and ½ inch wide. Lay these 1 inch apart on the prepared cookie sheet. Brush the bread sticks with the egg white, sprinkle with onion powder, and let them rise for 20 minutes in a warm place.

10. Preheat oven to 400° F.

11. Bake the bread sticks for 12 – 14 minutes, until nicely browned. Cool on cooking rack.

Yield: Makes 20 bread sticks

Each bread stick has approximately 41 calories, 1.6 g. protein, 0.2 g. total fat (0.1 g. unsaturated fat, 0 g. saturated fat), 8.4 g. carbohydrates, 0.1 mg. cholesterol, 0.7 g. fiber, 31 mg. sodium, 9.4 mg. calcium.

Exchanges per serving: ½ starch.

Jalapeño Corn Biscuits

The taste of these unusual biscuits is spicy and hot, the texture is coarse. It's a great combination.

½ cup plus 2 tablespoons
unbleached flour
½ cup plus 2 tablespoons
cornmeal
2 teaspoons baking powder
¼ teaspoon salt
1½ tablespoons chilled margarine, cut into 10 small pieces

¼ cup skim milk
¼ cup plain, low-fat yogurt
½ teaspoon chopped jalapeño or
fresh cayenne pepper
¼ cup grated part-skim mozzarella cheese

1. Preheat oven to 425° F. Lightly coat a baking sheet with nonstick cooking spray.

2. In a food processor combine the flour, cornmeal, baking powder, and salt, then add the chunks of margarine, and pulse the machine 5 or 6 times until the mixture is coarse and crumbly.

Or combine these dry ingredients in a bowl, and cut in the margarine with a pastry cutter or two forks to the same consistency.

3. Add the skim milk, yogurt, pepper, and cheese, and stir until the batter is moistened and pulls away from the sides of the bowl.

4. Transfer the batter to a lightly floured board, and knead the dough 5 or 6 times. Roll the dough out ¼ inch thick. Using a 1½-inch-diameter cookie cutter, cut the dough into 12 biscuits. You will have to reshape and reroll the scraps of dough a few times to utilize all the dough.

5. Place the rounds of dough on the prepared pan, and bake for 10 – 12 minutes, or until the biscuits are lightly browned.

Yield: Makes 12 biscuits

Each biscuit has approximately 71 calories, 2.3 g. protein, 2.5 g. total fat (1.4 g. unsaturated fat, 0.6 g. saturated fat), 10.5 g. carbohydrates, 1.4 mg. cholesterol, 1 g. fiber, 90 mg. sodium, 45 mg. calcium. Exchanges per serving: ½ fat, ⅔ starch.

Kasha Knishes

Envelopes of flaky pastry dough enclosing a fluffy kasha filling. We occasionally make it with Bulgur Pilaf (page 234), Wild and Brown Rice (page 231), and Lemon Couscous (page 236).

2⅔ cups of Speckled Kasha (page 237)
½ cup whole wheat flour
1 cup plus 2 tablespoons unbleached flour

1 teaspoon baking powder
½ cup skim milk
2 tablespoons oil
1 egg white, lightly beaten

1. Prepare the kasha, and set aside.
2. In a mixing bowl combine the whole wheat flour, 1 cup of the unbleached flour, and the baking powder.
3. In a measuring cup combine the milk and oil. Pour the liquid into the flour, and stir to form a stiff dough.
4. Sprinkle 1 tablespoon of the remaining flour on a pastry board or counter top. Knead the dough on the floured board for one minute. Place the dough in a small bowl, cover with plastic wrap, and refrigerate for 20 minutes.
5. Preheat oven to 400° F. Lightly coat a cookie sheet with non-stick cooking spray.
6. Dust your working surface with the remaining tablespoon of the flour. Transfer the dough to the floured area, cut it in half, then cut each half into 4 equal pieces.
7. Roll each piece out to a 4-inch square. Place ⅓ cup of the grain filling in the center of the dough. Fold one side of the dough over the filling, then the opposite side, then the other two sides to form a little packet, then pinch the dough in the center to seal the edges.
8. Place packets of dough on the prepared pan, brush them with beaten egg white, and bake for 15 minutes, until golden brown.

Yield: Makes 8 knishes

Each serving has approximately 133 calories, 4 g. protein, 3.8 g. total fat (3 g. unsaturated fat, 0.5 g. saturated fat), 21 g. carbohydrates, 0.3 mg. cholesterol, 1.5 g. fiber, 54 mg. sodium, 49 mg. calcium. Exchanges per serving: ⅔ fat, 1 starch, 1 vegetable.

Bagel Chips

Thin toasted buttery-tasting bagel rings to serve with dips.

2   **bagels (3-ounce size), each
    sliced into 7 rings**
1½ **tablespoons butter-flavored
    sprinkles**

2   **tablespoons water**
1   **teaspoon onion or garlic
    powder (optional)**

1. Preheat oven to 450° F. Lightly coat a large cookie sheet with non-stick cooking spray.
2. Spread the bagel rings in one layer on the prepared pan.
3. In a small bowl combine the butter sprinkles and water until well mixed.
4. With a pastry brush coat the top of the bagel rings with the butter-water. If you want onion- or garlic-flavored bagel chips, lightly sprinkle the flavored powders on top.
5. Bake for 12 minutes, until the tops are lightly brown and slightly crisp. Remove from oven, and let them sit for 5 minutes.

Yield: Makes 14 slices

Each slice has approximately 28 calories, 1 g. protein, 0.1 g. total fat (0 g. unsaturated fat, 0 g. saturated fat), 5.6 g. carbohydrates, 0 mg. cholesterol, 0.2 g. fiber, 101 mg. sodium, 2.9 mg. calcium.
Exchanges per serving: ⅓ starch.

Homemade Tortilla Chips

Crisp spicy chips to accompany Green Tomatillo Sauce (page 130) or Spicy Salsa (page 129).

3   **6-inch corn tortillas**
1   **teaspoon corn oil**
½   **teaspoon garlic powder**

½   **teaspoon onion powder**
½   **teaspoon chili powder**

1. Preheat oven to 400° F. Lightly coat a cookie sheet with non-stick cooking spray.
2. Cut each tortilla into 10 wedges.

3. Place the oil in a small bowl. Toss the chips in the oil, then lay them on the prepared cookie sheet.

4. Sprinkle the garlic, onion, and chili powders lightly over the chips, and bake for 7 minutes, until crisp.

Yield: Serves 4

Each 15-chip serving has approximately 62 calories, 1.6 g. protein, 2 g. total fat (1.2 g. unsaturated fat, 0.2 g. saturated fat), 10.4 g. carbohydrates, 0 mg. cholesterol, 2 g. fiber, 4 mg. sodium, 34 mg. calcium. Exchanges per serving: ⅓ fat, ⅔ starch.

Homemade Flour Tortillas with Scallions

These soft but slightly crisp tortillas taste much fresher than commercial ones, and they have the added bite of scallion bits.

1⅛–1¼ **cups unbleached flour**	½ **tablespoon corn oil**
⅓ **cup plus 1 tablespoon boiling water**	2 **tablespoons finely sliced scallions**

1. Place 1 cup of the flour in a mixing bowl, make a well in the center, add the water and oil, and stir to make a dough. Stir in the scallions.

2. Sprinkle a board with 1 tablespoon of the remaining flour, and knead the dough on it until smooth, about 8 minutes. Add more flour, a little at a time, if the dough gets too sticky.

3. Cut the dough into 8 equal pieces. On the lightly floured board roll each piece into a 5-inch circle with a rolling pin.

4. Pan-fry the tortillas, 3 at a time, in a cast-iron fry pan or griddle without oil for about 1 minute on each side, until lightly brown.

Yield: Makes 8 5-inch tortillas

Each tortilla has approximately 84 calories, 2.2 g. protein, 1 g. total fat (0.8 g. unsaturated fat, 0.1 g. saturated fat), 16 g. carbohydrates, 0 mg. cholesterol, 0.6 g. fiber, 0.5 mg. sodium, 4.2 mg. calcium. Exchanges per serving: 1 starch.

Corn Pancakes

Light springy pancakes dotted with chewy corn kernels. Serve with low-calorie maple syrup or topped with 21 Alarm Chili (page 192).

¾ cup unbleached flour	2 egg whites
½ cup whole-grain cornmeal	1 cup non-fat buttermilk
1 teaspoon baking powder	⅓ cup raw corn kernels
2 tablespoons sugar	

1. In a bowl combine the flour, cornmeal, baking powder, and sugar.

2. In a separate bowl, beat the egg whites, then add the buttermilk and corn. Mix these liquid ingredients into the dry ingredients, and stir until the dry ingredients are moistened.

3. Lightly coat a fry pan or griddle with non-stick cooking spray, and place over medium heat. When a drop of water dances on the hot surface, pour ¼ cup of batter into the pan or on the griddle for each pancake. Cook over medium-low heat until the top of the pancake bubbles, about 1–2 minutes, then flip each pancake over and cook until lightly brown on the second side, about 1 more minute. Transfer the cooked pancakes to a warm platter while you make the rest of the pancakes. Between batches, remove the pan from heat, re-spray with non-stick coating, and reheat the pan.

Yield: Makes 8 4-inch pancakes

Each pancake has approximately 99 calories, 4 g. protein, 0.6 g. total fat (0.4 g. unsaturated fat, 0.1 g. saturated fat), 20 g. carbohydrates, 0.5 mg. cholesterol, 1.4 g. fiber, 66 mg. sodium, 65 mg. calcium. Exchanges per serving: 1¼ starch.

Blintzes

These are Russian-style crepes filled with sweetened cheese. Have them for breakfast or dinner, or lunch, for that matter.

2 cups low-fat (1%) cottage cheese	4 teaspoons sugar
2 teaspoons grated lemon peel	8 Perfect Crepes (page 265)
½ teaspoon cinnamon	2 teaspoons margarine

1. In a bowl combine cottage cheese, lemon peel, cinnamon, and sugar for the filling.

2. Place ¼ cup of the cheese filling in the center of each crepe. Fold the top and bottom down over the filling, then fold over the two sides to form a square packet.

3. Preheat a non-stick fry pan or griddle, and melt 1 teaspoon of the margarine. Place 4 blintzes on the hot pan, seam side down, and cook on medium-low heat for about 2 minutes, until lightly browned. Lower the heat and carefully turn the blintzes over with a spatula, then cook for 2 more minutes. Transfer the blintzes to a warm plate. Repeat the procedure for the remaining blintzes. Serve immediately.

Yield: Makes 8 blintzes

Each blintz has approximately 125 calories, 9.5 g. protein, 3.1 g. total fat (2.1 g. unsaturated fat, 0.9 g. saturated fat), 14.4 g. carbohydrates, 2.5 mg. cholesterol, 0.8 g. fiber, 337 mg. sodium, 42 mg. calcium. Exchanges per serving: ½ fat, ½ milk, ¾ starch.

Blueberry Oatmeal Pancakes

Tender pancakes flecked with fresh blueberries. Serve with low-calorie syrup or a dollop of Creamy Yogurt Cheese (page 124).

½ tablespoon margarine	¼ cup unbleached flour
⅔ cup skim milk	¼ cup whole wheat flour
1 egg white	½ tablespoon baking powder
1 cup blueberries	⅛ teaspoon salt
¼ cup rolled oats	1 tablespoon sugar

1. Melt the margarine in a small pan.

2. In a bowl combine the milk, egg white, and blueberries with the melted margarine.

3. In a separate bowl combine the rolled oats, unbleached and whole wheat flours, baking powder, salt, and sugar. Add the blueberry-milk mixture to the dry ingredients and mix well.

4. Lightly coat a 10-inch non-stick griddle or fry pan with non-stick cooking spray. Heat it over medium heat until a few drops of water sizzle.

5. Using a ¼-cup measure, pour 3 or 4 pancakes on the hot griddle. Cook over medium-low heat for about 1 minute, until the pancake

tops bubble and their edges become firm. Flip each pancake over with a spatula, and continue cooking for 1 more minute. Transfer the pancakes to a warm plate. Remove the griddle from heat, coat again with non-stick cooking spray, and repeat until you have used all the batter.

Yield: Makes 8 pancakes

Each pancake has approximately 69 calories, 2.6 g. protein, 1 g. total fat (0.8 g. unsaturated fat, 0.2 g. saturated fat), 13 g. carbohydrates, 0.4 mg. cholesterol, 1.4 g. fiber, 122 mg. sodium, 41 mg. calcium. Exchanges per serving: ¼ fat, ⅛ fruit, ⅔ starch.

Perfect Crepes

1 tablespoon margarine	¼ teaspoon salt
⅔ cup unbleached flour	2 egg whites
¼ cup whole wheat flour	10 ounces skim milk

1. Melt the margarine, and set aside.
2. In a medium-sized mixing bowl, combine the unbleached and whole wheat flours and salt.
3. In a separate mixing bowl whisk the egg whites lightly, and stir in the milk and melted margarine. Pour this into the dry ingredients, and stir well until the batter is free of lumps.
4. Lightly coat an 8-inch non-stick fry pan with non-stick cooking spray, and heat it over medium heat. Pour in a scant ¼ cup of batter. Tilt the pan slightly and quickly to let batter completely coat the bottom of the pan, and pour any excess batter back into the bowl.
5. Cook the crepe for 40 seconds, until it solidifies, browns slightly at the edges, and bubbles on top. Quickly flip the crepe over with a spatula suitable for the non-stick surface, and cook for 20 seconds. Carefully transfer the crepe to a warm plate. Repeat the process until all the batter is used, recoating the crepe pan each time with non-stick cooking spray.

Yield: Makes 8 crepes

Each crepe has approximately 67 calories, 2.4 g. protein, 1.6 g. total fat (1.2 g. unsaturated fat, 0.3 g. saturated fat), 10.6 g. carbohydrates, 0 mg. cholesterol, 0.8 g. fiber, 96.2 mg. sodium, 5.1 mg. calcium. Exchanges per serving: ¼ fat, ⅔ starch.

Desserts

Fresh Berry Tart
Peach Crisp
Pumpkin Pie
Perfect Pie Crust
Strawberry Rhubarb Pie
Key Lime Pie
Blueberry Cream Cheese Pie
Strawberry Crepes
Apple Strudel
Baked Apples with Rasp-
   berries and Cognac
Poached Pears in Cranberry
   Glaze
Broiled Grapefruit
Figs in a Chocolate Pool
Exotic Fresh Fruits with
   Mango Cream

Chocolate Cake
Chocolate Brownies
Applesauce Cake
Chocolate Meringue Cake
Butterscotch Squares
Poppy Seed Cookies with
   Raspberry Jam
Apricot Oat Bran Cookies
Caramel Popcorn
Mocha Mousse
Fruity Couscous Pudding
Chocolate-Covered Bananas
Raspberry Creme
Frozen Strawberry Sorbet
Mango Sorbet
Fruity Frozen Yogurt Pops
Orange Cream Pops

Fresh Berry Tart

Glistening fresh fruit on a crunchy base. We often substitute (or add) blueberries.

Crust:

¾ cup (3 ounces) wheat and barley nugget cereal (like Nutri-Grain or Grapenuts), finely ground in a blender or food processor
¾ cup graham cracker crumbs
1 tablespoon brown sugar
½ cup water

Filling:

1½ cups part-skim ricotta cheese
1½ cups low-fat (1%) cottage cheese

¼ cup skim milk
1 envelope unflavored gelatin
3 packets non-nutritive sweetener

Fruit topping:

½ cup reduced-sugar apricot jam
1 tablespoon water
½ pint strawberries or raspberries
1 kiwi fruit

1. Preheat oven to 350° F.

2. In a 10-inch springform pan, combine the crust ingredients and mix until lumpy. Using fingertips, press the crust into the bottom of the pan. Bake for 10 minutes, and remove from oven.

3. In a food processor or blender lightly puree the ricotta and cottage cheeses.

4. In a small saucepan combine the milk and gelatin. Let it sit off the heat for 1–2 minutes, then warm over low heat, stirring until the gelatin dissolves. Remove from heat, stir in the sweetener, and combine with the cheeses. Pour the filling over the crust, and refrigerate for 1 hour.

5. In a small saucepan heat the apricot jam with the water over very low heat. When the jam thins out, after 1 to 2 minutes, remove from heat and set aside.

6. Place halved strawberries or whole raspberries ½ inch apart around the inside rim of the pan. Peel the kiwi, cut it into thin slices, and arrange in a circle 1 inch inside the berries. Add another circle of berries 1 inch inside the kiwi. Using a pastry brush or spoon, lightly spread a thin layer of warm apricot jam over the fruit. Refrigerate until serving.

Yield: Serves 10

Each serving has approximately 162 calories, 10.8 g. protein, 4.3 g. total fat (1.8 g. unsaturated fat, 2.3 g. saturated fat), 20.6 g. carbohydrates, 12.9 mg. cholesterol, 1.5 g. fiber, 300 mg. sodium, 134 mg. calcium.

Exchanges per serving: ¼ fruit, ¾ milk, 1 starch.

Peach Crisp

A crumbly topping over juicy peaches.

3 large peaches, peeled and sliced	1 teaspoon cinnamon
2 tablespoons cornstarch	2 tablespoons cold water
1 tablespoon sugar	1 tablespoon brown sugar
	1 tablespoon margarine

Topping:

½ cup rolled oats
¼ cup (1 ounce) wheat nugget
cereal (like Grapenuts or
Nutri-Grain)

1. Preheat oven to 375° F. Coat a 6×8-inch pie pan with non-stick cooking spray.
2. Mix the peach slices with the cornstarch and sugar until the cornstarch is invisible.
3. In a food processor, process the topping ingredients until the mixture is moist and lumpy.
4. Spoon the peaches into the pie pan, cover with the topping, and bake for 25 minutes. Serve warm.

Yield: Serves 4

Each serving has approximately 158 calories, 3 g. protein, 3.6 g. total fat (2.8 g. unsaturated fat, 0.7 g. saturated fat), 30.2 g. carbohydrates, 0 mg. cholesterol, 2.9 g. fiber, 84.7 mg. sodium, 22 mg. calcium.

Exchanges per serving: ¾ fat, ¾ fruit, 1 starch.

Pumpkin Pie

This is lighter and creamier than other pumpkin pies, with rich earthy spices.

¾ cup graham cracker crumbs	1 teaspoon ground cinnamon
3 tablespoons water	⅛ teaspoon ground nutmeg
1 box (1.9-ounce) sugar-free instant vanilla pudding	⅛ teaspoon allspice
2 cups skim milk	¼ teaspoon ground ginger
¾ cup canned pumpkin meat, pureed	¼ teaspoon rum extract

1. Preheat oven to 350° F. Lightly coat an 8-inch pie pan with non-stick cooking spray.

2. Combine the graham cracker crumbs and water in a food processor until moistened.

3. Press the crumbs into the bottom (not sides) of the prepared pie pan, and bake for 8 minutes.

4. In a 1-quart saucepan combine the pudding mix and milk and cook until the mixture comes to a boil. Stir in the pumpkin puree, the spices, and the rum extract.

5. Pour the filling into the baked graham cracker crust, and refrigerate until set.

Yield: Serves 8

Each serving has approximately 89 calories, 3.2 g. protein, 1.4 g. total fat (0.8 g. unsaturated fat, 0.4 g. saturated fat), 16.3 g. carbohydrates, 1 mg. cholesterol, 0.8 g. fiber, 172 mg. sodium, 89 mg. calcium. Exchanges per serving: ⅛ milk, ⅞ starch.

Perfect Pie Crust

A flaky pie shell for many recipes, among them Strawberry Rhubarb Pie (page 271).

½ cup plus 2 tablespoons all-purpose unbleached flour
¼ cup whole wheat flour
3 tablespoons cold margarine, cut into small pieces

3–4 tablespoons ice water
2 cups dried beans, washed, or pie weights

1. Preheat oven to 450° F. Lightly coat an 8-inch pie pan with non-stick cooking spray.

2. Combine ½ cup of the unbleached flour with the whole wheat flour in a bowl, or in a food processor bowl, and add the margarine.

3. In the bowl, use a fork to crumble the flour and margarine into a coarse mixture. In the food processor, use the metal chopping blade and pulse the machine 10–12 times to cut the margarine into small pieces. As you form the mixture, add the ice water, 1 tablespoon at a time, until the lumps appear moist.

4. Transfer the dough to a board, and lightly knead it for 1 minute. Form into a ball, place in a small bowl, cover with plastic wrap, and refrigerate for 10 minutes.

5. Sprinkle the remaining 2 tablespoons of flour on a pastry board and lightly coat the rolling pin with flour. On the floured board roll the pie dough out in a circle slightly larger than your pie pan. Carefully transfer the dough to the prepared pie pan. Crimp the edges of the dough against the rim of the pie pan. You can use this unbaked pie shell in many recipes, except with fruit fillings.

6. If you are making a fruit-filled pie, you must pre-bake the shell so the fruit juices won't make it soggy. To pre-bake it, cover the crust with tinfoil, place 2 cups of clean beans or pie weights in the center of the crust, and bake for 10 minutes.

Yield: Makes 1 8-inch pie shell serving 8

Each serving of crust has approximately 79 calories, 1.4 g. protein, 4.4 g. total fat (3.3 g. unsaturated fat, 0.9 g. saturated fat), 8.7 g. carbohydrates, 0 mg. cholesterol, 0.7 g. fiber, 50 mg. sodium, 4.4 mg. calcium.

Exchanges per serving: ½ fat, ¾ starch.

Strawberry Rhubarb Pie

Sweet berries and chewy, tart rhubarb in a flaky crust.

1 **Perfect Pie Crust (see page 270), pre-baked**	3½ **tablespoons cornstarch**
2½ **cups rhubarb, cut into 1-inch slices**	¼ **cup juice from frozen strawberries or water**
3 **cups fresh or frozen unsweetened strawberries, defrosted**	⅓ **cup sugar**

1. Preheat oven heat to 450° F.
2. Make the pre-baked pie crust.
3. In a bowl combine the rhubarb, strawberries, cornstarch, water or juice, and sugar. Mix well to coat the fruit with cornstarch and sugar, then let sit for 10 minutes.
4. Fill the pre-baked pie shell with the fruit mixture. Cover the edges of the crust with foil to prevent browning. Bake for 10 minutes at 450° F., then reduce heat to 350°, and continue baking for 25 to 30 minutes. Remove the pie from the oven and let it cool to room temperature before serving.

Yield: Serves 8

Each serving has approximately 149 calories, 2.1 g. protein, 4.7 g. total fat (3.6 g. unsaturated fat, 0.9 g. saturated fat), 25.6 g. carbohydrates, 0 mg. cholesterol, 3.2 g. fiber, 53 mg. sodium, 66 mg. calcium. Exchanges per serving: ½ fat, 1 fruit, 1¼ starch.

Key Lime Pie

Tart citrus pie topped with creamy meringue.

¾ **cup graham cracker crumbs**	1½ **teaspoons grated lime peel**
2–3 **tablespoons water**	1½ **cups skim milk**
1 **package sugar-free vanilla pudding mix (not instant)**	3 **egg whites**
7 **tablespoons lime or key lime juice**	¼ **teaspoon cream of tartar**
	1½ **tablespoons sugar**

1. Preheat oven to 350° F. Lightly coat an 8-inch pie plate with non-stick cooking spray.

2. In a bowl, combine graham cracker crumbs and water until crumbly. Press the crumbs against the bottom and sides of the prepared pie plate, and bake for 10 minutes. Remove from oven, and let cool.

3. In a saucepan combine the pudding mix, lime juice, and lime peel, gradually whisk in the milk, and cook over medium heat, stirring, until the mixture comes to a boil and thickens.

Or combine all ingredients in the same way in a 1½ quart microwave-safe bowl, and cook on high, uncovered, for 6 minutes, stirring the mixture after 3 minutes.

Pour the thickened pudding into the baked pie shell.

4. In a medium-sized mixing bowl beat the egg whites with an electric beater until they form soft peaks, then add the cream of tartar and sugar, and continue beating until the whites are stiff.

5. Carefully spread the beaten egg whites over the pie, and bake for 10 minutes, until lightly browned. Remove from the oven and let cool, then refrigerate until serving.

Yield: Serves 8

Each serving has approximately 93 calories, 3.7 g. protein, 1.3 g. total fat (0.8 g. unsaturated fat, 0.4 g. saturated fat), 17 g. carbohydrates, 0.8 mg. cholesterol, 0.4 g. fiber, 182 mg. sodium, 65 mg. calcium. Exchanges per serving: ⅕ milk, ¾ starch.

Blueberry Cream Cheese Pie

Yes, a low-fat cream cheese pie, and it's creamy and fruity.

1 **Perfect Pie Shell (page 270), pre-baked**	1 **egg**
1½ **cups low-fat (1%) cottage cheese**	2 **cups fresh or unsweetened frozen blueberries, defrosted**
4 **tablespoons sugar**	3 **tablespoons cornstarch**

1. Preheat oven to 450° F.

2. Make the pre-baked pie crust.

3. In the food processor, combine the cottage cheese, 2 tablespoons of the sugar, and the egg until smooth. Pour into the bottom of the

partially baked pie shell, and bake for 10 minutes. Remove from oven, reduce heat to 350°. Cover the pie crust edge with foil to prevent browning.

4. In a bowl stir together the blueberries, remaining 2 tablespoons of sugar, and cornstarch. Let sit for 10 minutes. Pour over the cheese mixture, and bake for 25 minutes. Let cool to room temperature, then refrigerate until serving.

Yield: Serves 10
Each serving has approximately 140 calories, 6.1 g. protein, 4.5 g. total fat (3.2 g. unsaturated fat, 1.1 g. saturated fat), 19 g. carbohydrates, 22.3 mg. cholesterol, 1.4 g. fiber, 187 mg. sodium, 29 mg. calcium. Exchanges per serving: ½ fruit, ⅓ milk, 1 starch.

Strawberry Crepes

You can gild these deceptively sweet and rich-tasting crepes with a dollop of Raspberry Sauce (page 139) or serve them up for an elegant breakfast or brunch.

¼ cup whole wheat flour	½ teaspoon orange extract
2 tablespoons unbleached flour	1 pint fresh strawberries (about
¼ teaspoon salt	1½ cups)
2 egg whites	4 teaspoons confectioners sugar
½ cup skim milk	

1. In a bowl combine the whole wheat and unbleached flours, salt, egg whites, milk, and flavor extract. Mix well with a whisk.

2. Lightly coat an 8-inch non-stick pan with non-stick cooking spray. Heat the pan on medium-high heat. When a drop of water dances on the hot surface, pour a scant ¼ cup of batter into the pan, tilting it gently to spread the batter evenly. Cook the crepe for 1 minute on each side, then remove the crepe and place it on a paper towel. Take the pan off the heat, respray it, and reheat it for 10 seconds. Add enough batter to make another crepe, and repeat the procedure until all the batter is used.

3. Set aside four whole unblemished strawberries for a garnish. Remove the stems from the remaining berries and cut them into small pieces.

4. Spoon ¼ cup of the cut strawberries onto one end of each crepe.

Roll the crepe lengthwise to form a cylinder. Place the crepes seam side down on a serving platter, dust each one with 1 teaspoon of confectioners sugar, and garnish with a strawberry.

Yield: Makes 4 crepes

Each crepe has approximately 83 calories, 4.5 g. protein, 0.5 g. total fat (0.3 g. unsaturated fat, 0.1 g. saturated fat), 16 g. carbohydrates, 0.5 mg. cholesterol, 2.5 g. fiber, 175 mg. sodium, 52 mg. calcium. Exchanges per serving: ¾ fruit, ½ starch.

Apple Strudel

Flaky dough wrapped around spiced apples and bits of dates.

2 cups Rome or Granny Smith apples, peeled and thinly sliced (½ pound)	¼ teaspoon nutmeg
	1 tablespoon finely chopped dates
1 tablespoon lemon juice	1 teaspoon cornstarch
1 tablespoon apple juice concentrate	2 teaspoons margarine
	2 sheets phyllo dough
1 teaspoon cinnamon	

1. Preheat oven to 375° F. Lightly coat a cookie sheet with non-stick cooking spray.

2. In a medium-sized bowl combine the sliced apples, lemon juice, apple juice concentrate, cinnamon, nutmeg, dates, and cornstarch.

3. Melt the margarine. On a dry counter lay one sheet of phyllo dough on top of the other with a short side facing you, and lightly brush the top surface with a little melted margarine.

4. Drain and reserve the fruit juices, and pile the apple-date mixture across the lower width of the phyllo dough, about an inch in from the bottom edge. Carefully roll the phyllo dough away from you into a tight roll encasing the apples. With a spatula carefully transfer the roll to the prepared pan, seam side down. Brush the top and sides of the phyllo dough with the remaining margarine to seal, then brush with the reserved juices for extra flavor, and bake for 30 minutes, or until brown.

Yield: Makes 8 1-inch slices

Each slice has approximately 43 calories, 0.4 g. protein, 1.2 g. total fat (0.8 g. unsaturated fat, 0.2 g. saturated fat), 8.6 g. carbohydrates, 0 mg. cholesterol, 0.8 g. fiber, 23 mg. sodium, 6 mg. calcium. Exchanges per serving: ¼ fat, ½ fruit.

Baked Apples with Raspberries and Cognac

Deep raspberry flavor buried in the heart of a tender apple.

4 small Rome apples	2 tablespoons cognac
1½ cups fresh or sugar-free frozen raspberries, defrosted	2 teaspoons brown sugar

1. Core the apples halfway, then peel the apples halfway down from the top.

2. In a bowl, mix the raspberries, cognac, and brown sugar. Spoon into the cored apples.

3. Cook according to either method:

To bake in the oven, preheat oven to 375° F. Place the apples in an oven-proof dish, cover, and bake for 20 minutes, turning the dish in the oven after 10 minutes. If the apples aren't tender, bake for 5 more minutes.

To microwave, place the apples in a microwave-safe dish, cover tightly with plastic wrap, and cook on high for 2 minutes; rotate the dish 180 degrees (unless your microwave has a revolving turntable) and cook on high for an additional 2 minutes. Pierce with a fork to test for tenderness. If the apples are not tender, cook for another minute or two. Note that the apples will continue cooking after you remove them from the microwave, and that they will fall apart in the microwave if overcooked.

4. Spoon any excess raspberry sauce in the bottom of the pan over the apples.

Yield: Serves 4

Each serving has approximately 127 calories, 0.7 g. protein, 0.7 g. total fat (0.3 g. unsaturated fat, 0.1 g. saturated fat), 28.5 g. carbohydrates, 0 mg. cholesterol, 6.3 g. fiber, 2 mg. sodium, 22 mg. calcium. Exchanges per serving: 2 fruit.

Poached Pears in Cranberry Glaze

Sweet, tender pears in a tangy, viscous, cranberry glaze.

4 ripe, medium-size D'Anjou pears, peeled and cored	½ cup apple juice concentrate
1 cup water	1 cup cranberries, rinsed and picked over

1. Combine the ingredients in 1½ quart pot, bring to a boil, then reduce to a simmer and cook, uncovered, for 7 minutes. Turn the pears over, and continue cooking until they are fork-tender, about 15 minutes in all.

2. Remove the pears from the pot, let cool, cut in half lengthwise, and set aside.

3. Drain the liquid and cranberries through a fine-mesh strainer, reserving the liquid. Puree the cranberries in a blender or food processor, then add the strained liquid and puree a second time. You should have about 1 cup.

4. To serve, pour about 2 tablespoons of cranberry sauce on each serving plate, and place the pear in the center.

Yield: Serves 8
Each serving has approximately 94.8 calories, 0.5 g. protein, 0.42 g. total fat (0.24 g. unsaturated fat, 0.04 g. saturated fat), 23.7 g. carbohydrates, 0 mg. cholesterol, 3.3 g. fiber, 4.6 mg. sodium, 15.5 mg. calcium.
Exchanges per serving: 1½ fruit.

Broiled Grapefruit

Slightly sweet and spicy version of a familiar low-cal stand-by dressed up for dessert.

½ grapefruit	⅛ teaspoon ground nutmeg
½ teaspoon brown sugar	

1. Preheat broiler.

2. Free each grapefruit section from its surrounding membrane with a sharp paring knife.

3. Mix the brown sugar and nutmeg together, then sprinkle over the top of the grapefruit.

4. Broil for 2 minutes.

Yield: Serves 1

Each serving has approximately 46 calories, 0.7 g. protein, 0.1 g. total fat (0.05 g. unsaturated fat, 0.02 g. saturated fat), 11.7 g. carbohydrates, 0 mg. cholesterol, 1.6 g. fiber, 1.01 mg. sodium, 14.9 mg. calcium.
Exchanges per serving: ¾ fruit.

Figs in a Chocolate Pool

Chewy figs and smooth chocolate make an excellent combination, but you can substitute strawberries, pineapple, orange sections, pear slices, or another favorite fruit.

4 tablespoons unsweetened cocoa powder	6 packets non-nutritive sweetener
½ cup cold skim milk	4 fresh figs, cut into eighths
	8 mint leaves for garnish

1. In a small saucepan or microwave-safe bowl stir the cocoa and milk together until free of lumps.

2. Heat the mixture on the range over low heat or microwave for 1 minute on high, covered, stirring the chocolate mixture until smooth. Stir in the sweetener.

3. Pour one-fourth of the chocolate sauce into the center of four dessert plates, and arrange the fig slices like spokes around the chocolate pool, so that half of each fig slice sits in the chocolate. Garnish each plate with mint leaves.

Yield: Serves 4

Each serving has approximately 68 calories, 2.4 g. protein, 1.2 g. total fat (0.5 g. unsaturated fat, 0.7 g. saturated fat), 15.2 g. carbohydrates, 0.5 mg. cholesterol, 3.5 g. fiber, 18 mg. sodium, 64 mg. calcium.
Exchanges per serving: ¼ fat, ⅔ fruit, ⅛ milk, ⅛ starch.

Exotic Fresh Fruits with Mango Cream

Beautifully arranged cool and refreshing fruits served with a creamy tropical sauce.

1 tablespoon lemon juice	1 starfruit, cut into 8 slices
2 cups cold water	1 kiwi fruit, peeled and sliced
1 Asian pear	½ cup fresh raspberries
1 papaya, cut in half, seeded, then each half quartered	1 cup Mango Cream Sauce (page 139)

1. In a bowl combine the lemon juice and water. Slice the pear vertically into quarters, remove the core, cut each quarter into 4 thin slices, and transfer the 16 pear slices to the bowl.

2. Arrange the papaya slices on a serving platter like 8 spokes of a wheel. At the rim of the platter between each slice of papaya, place a slice of starfruit.

3. Arrange the kiwi, raspberries, and drained pear slices decoratively around the other fruits. Serve Mango Cream Sauce on the side.

Yield: Serves 8

Each serving has approximately 62 calories, 0.9 g. protein, 0.4 g. total fat (0.2 g. unsaturated fat, 0 g. saturated fat), 15.6 g. carbohydrates, 0.1 mg. cholesterol, 3.2 g. fiber, 5 mg. sodium, 27 mg. calcium. Exchanges per serving: 1 fruit.

Chocolate Cake

Yes, chocolate cake, with a nice chocolate flavor and a tender crumb.

3 tablespoons margarine	¼ teaspoon salt
½ cup sugar	1 teaspoon baking soda
1 egg	1 teaspoon baking powder
1¼ cups non-fat buttermilk	1½ cups unbleached flour, sifted
¼ cup unsweetened cocoa powder	

1. Preheat oven to 375° F. Lightly coat an 8-inch round cake pan with non-stick cooking spray.

2. With an electric mixer cream the margarine and sugar in a mixing bowl. Beat in the egg.

3. Stir in the buttermilk. Set the bowl aside.

4. In a large bowl, combine the cocoa, salt, baking soda, baking powder, and flour, and mix together well.

5. Add the creamed margarine–buttermilk mixture to the dry ingredients in one batch. Stir until the dry ingredients are thoroughly moistened.

6. Pour the batter into the prepared pan and smooth the top with a spatula. Bake for 35 minutes, or until a cake tester comes out dry. Remove from the pan and let cool on a rack.

Yield: Makes 12 servings
Each serving has approximately 130 calories, 3.3 g. protein, 3.8 g. total fat (2.6 g. unsaturated fat, 0.9 g. saturated fat), 21.5 g. carbohydrates, 17.8 mg. cholesterol, 0.9 g. fiber, 190 mg. sodium, 55.2 mg. calcium. Exchanges per serving: ½ fat, 1⅓ starch.

Chocolate Brownies

For chocolate fans, these are about as low-cal as nutty brownies can get, and still keep their rich, chocolate flavor and crunch.

2½ tablespoons margarine, softened	1 egg
⅓ cup sugar	½ cup less one tablespoon sifted, unbleached flour
¼ cup unsweetened cocoa powder	1½ tablespoons chopped walnuts

1. Preheat oven to 350° F. Lightly coat a 3½×7½-inch loaf pan with non-stick cooking spray.

2. With an electric mixer, cream the margarine and sugar in a 1-quart bowl. Stir in the cocoa powder, then add the egg and blend on low for 30 seconds, scrape sides, and continue blending for 30 seconds more.

3. Sift in the flour, and stir until well incorporated. Stir in the nuts. Spread the batter evenly into the prepared pan. Bake for 18 minutes, or until a cake tester comes out slightly moist. Cool, then cut into 10 squares.

Yield: Makes 10 1½-inch brownies

Each piece has approximately 91 calories, 1.9 g. protein, 4.5 g. total fat (3.2 g. unsaturated fat, 1 g. saturated fat), 12 g. carbohydrates, 20.8 mg. cholesterol, 0.8 g. fiber, 40.8 mg. sodium, 8.4 mg. calcium. Exchanges per serving: 1 fat, ½ starch.

Applesauce Cake

Spiced with nutmeg and cloves, and dotted with raisins, this is a sweet cake with a rich flavor and a tender crumb.

3 tablespoons margarine, softened	1½ teaspoons cinnamon
⅓ cup molasses	¼ teaspoon salt
¼ cup brown sugar	1 teaspoon baking powder
1 egg	1 teaspoon baking soda
1 cup sugar-free applesauce	⅓ cup raisins
½ cup low-fat or non-fat buttermilk	1¾ cups unbleached flour, sifted
	¼ teaspoon nutmeg
	¼ teaspoon cloves

1. Preheat oven to 375° F. Coat an 8-inch square baking pan with non-stick vegetable spray.

2. In a bowl, combine the margarine with the molasses, brown sugar, and egg. Mix until smooth. Stir in the applesauce and buttermilk.

3. In another bowl, combine the remaining ingredients. Add the wet ingredients to the dry ingredients, stirring until the dry ingredients are well moistened.

4. Pour the batter in the prepared pan. Bake for 35 minutes, or until a toothpick or cake tester comes out clean.

Yield: Makes 12 servings

Each serving has approximately 141 calories, 3 g. protein, 3.5 g. total fat (2.5 g. unsaturated fat, 0.77 g. saturated fat), 24.7 g. carbohydrates, 17.5 mg. cholesterol, 1.1 g. fiber, 185 mg. sodium, 44.6 mg. calcium. Exchanges per serving: ½ fat, ½ fruit, 1 starch.

Chocolate Meringue Cake

An airy, springy cake with the light touch of chocolate. Serve it with ices or Raspberry Sauce (page 139).

⅞	cup all-purpose flour	1⅓	cups egg whites (about 10 or
4	tablespoons unsweetened		11 eggs), at room temperature
	cocoa powder	½	teaspoon salt
1	cup sugar	1	teaspoon chocolate extract
1	teaspoon baking powder	1	teaspoon cream of tartar

1. Preheat the oven to 350° F. Have a clean, dry angel food pan ready.

2. Chill a large mixing bowl or the bowl from your electric mixer in the freezer for 15 minutes.

3. Sift together the flour, cocoa, ¼ cup of the sugar, and the baking powder 5 times. Set aside.

4. Add the egg whites to the chilled mixing bowl and beat with an electric mixer until they are white and slightly thickened, about 2 minutes. Add the salt, chocolate extract, and cream of tartar, and beat for 2 more minutes. Slowly add the remaining ¾ cup of sugar and continue to beat about 2 or 3 minutes, or until the egg whites are thick but slightly moist, with small peaks that fold over.

5. Sift the flour mixture a little at a time over the beaten egg whites. Each time fold the flour lightly into the egg whites with a whisk and not an electric mixer, being careful to preserve the airy volume of the egg whites.

6. Carefully pour the batter into the angel food pan. Bake for 30–35 minutes, or until the top of the cake feels dry.

7. Remove the cake from the oven and turn the pan upside down over an inverted funnel. Let the cake rest upside down for 1½ hours. Turn right side up, cut around the inside of the pan to free the cake, and remove the bottom of the pan.

Yield: Serves 10

Each serving has approximately 139 calories, 5 g. protein, 0.5 g. total fat (0.2 g. unsaturated fat, 0.3 g. saturated fat), 30 g. carbohydrates, 0 mg. cholesterol, 0.9 g. fiber, 187 mg. sodium, 28 mg. calcium. Exchanges per serving: ⅓ meat, 1½ starch.

Butterscotch Squares

Think butterscotch brownies.

3 tablespoons margarine, softened
¼ cup brown sugar
1 egg

1 teaspoon vanilla
⅓ cup plus 2 tablespoons sifted, unbleached flour

1. Preheat oven to 350° F. Lightly coat a 3½×7½-inch baking pan with non-stick cooking spray.
2. Cream the margarine and brown sugar together with an electric mixer. Mix in the egg and vanilla. Stir in the flour until combined.
3. Spread the batter in the prepared pan, and bake for 15 minutes.
4. Cool and cut into 10 squares.

Yield: Makes 10 1½-inch squares

Each square has approximately 78 calories, 1.3 g. protein, 0.4 g. total fat (2.9 g. unsaturated fat, 0.9 g. saturated fat), 9.6 g. carbohydrates, 21 mg. cholesterol, 0.2 g. fiber, 49 mg. sodium, 9 mg. calcium. Exchanges per serving: ¾ fat, ½ starch.

Poppy Seed Cookies with Raspberry Jam

Sweet butter cookies flecked with poppy seeds and topped with a dollop of jam.

¼ cup margarine, softened
¼ cup sugar
1 egg
½ teaspoon vanilla
1¼ cups plus 3 tablespoons unbleached flour

1 teaspoon poppy seeds
1 teaspoon baking powder
¼ teaspoon salt
1 tablespoon low-sugar raspberry jam

1. In a bowl cream together the margarine and sugar with an electric beater until fluffy. Add the egg and vanilla, and beat for 10 more seconds.
2. In a separate bowl, combine 1¼ cups of the flour, the poppy seeds, baking powder, and salt. Slowly add the dry ingredients to the margarine mixture, stirring to form a stiff dough.

3. Sprinkle 1 tablespoon of the remaining flour on a pastry board, and knead the dough for 1 minute. Divide the dough in half, and place both halves in a small bowl, cover with plastic wrap, and refrigerate for 1 hour.

4. Preheat oven to 375° F. Lightly coat a cookie sheet with non-stick cooking spray.

5. Dust a pastry board with 1 tablespoon of the remaining flour, and lay half the dough on it. Cut the dough into 3 pieces, then cut each third into 4 pieces. With your palms roll each piece into a small ball. Place the 12 balls of dough on the prepared cookie sheet about 1½ inches apart. Press lightly on the top of each ball with a finger to make a small indentation, and into each place about ¼ teaspoon of the raspberry jam. Repeat the procedure for the remaining half of the dough. Bake for 12 minutes.

Yield: Makes 24 1½-inch cookies

Each cookie has approximately 54 calories, 1 g. protein, 2.2 g. total fat (1.7 g. unsaturated fat, 0.5 g. saturated fat), 7.4 g. carbohydrates, 8.7 mg. cholesterol, 0.2 g. fiber, 60 mg. sodium, 12 mg. calcium. Exchanges per serving: ⅓ fat, ½ starch.

Apricot Oat Bran Cookies

Butter cookies studded with bits of chewy apricots.

3 tablespoons margarine, softened	½ cup unbleached flour
	⅓ cup oat bran
3 tablespoons brown sugar	½ teaspoon baking soda
½ teaspoon vanilla extract	¼ teaspoon salt
2 egg whites	¼ cup chopped dried apricots

1. Preheat oven to 375° F. Lightly coat a cookie sheet with non-stick cooking spray.

2. In a bowl, cream the margarine and brown sugar with an electric mixer. Stir in the vanilla and egg whites. Set aside.

3. In a separate bowl, combine the remaining ingredients. Stir them into the margarine mixture and combine well.

4. Drop the dough, about 2 teaspoons at a time, on the prepared cookie sheet, and bake for 12 minutes, until the edges start to brown.

Yield: Makes about 18 2-inch cookies

Each cookie has approximately 45 calories, 1.1 g. protein, 2 g. total fat (1.5 g. unsaturated fat, 0.4 g. saturated fat), 6.4 g. carbohydrates, 0 mg. cholesterol, 0.4 g. fiber, 82 mg. sodium, 5.2 mg. calcium. Exchanges per serving: ⅓ fat, ⅓ starch.

Caramel Popcorn

Sweet, crunchy, chewy — a treat.

½ **cup raw popping corn**
5 **ounces water**
2 **tablespoons brown sugar**

   1. Pop corn in a hot-air popcorn popper or in a microwave popcorn popper according to manufacturer's instructions. You will make about 11 cups of popcorn.

   2. In a 1½-quart saucepan bring the sugar and water to a boil. Reduce to a simmer and cook for 10 minutes, or until the mixture thickens. Remove from heat immediately and quickly pour over the popcorn, stirring continuously.

Yield: Makes 11 cups

Each 1-cup serving has approximately 39 calories, 1 g. protein, 0.4 g. total fat (0.3 g. unsaturated fat, 0.1 g. saturated fat), 8.4 g. carbohydrates, 0 mg. cholesterol, 1.3 g. fiber, 1.6 mg. sodium, 3.1 mg. calcium. Exchanges per serving: ½ starch.

Mocha Mousse

A creamy, light, and airy mousse with minimal calories and fat. It's quick and easy in a microwave.

2½ tablespoons cornstarch
2 cups skim milk
3 tablespoons unsweetened cocoa powder
1½ tablespoons instant coffee
1 egg yolk, lightly beaten

6 packets non-nutritive sweetener
2 egg whites, at room temperature
¼ teaspoon cream of tartar

To cook on the range:

1. Mix the cornstarch and ½ cup of the milk in a small bowl, and set aside.

2. In a heavy 2-quart saucepan combine the cocoa, instant coffee, and the remaining 1½ cups of milk, and heat over medium-low heat, stirring constantly to dissolve the cocoa. Stir the cornstarch into the warm cocoa mixture, stirring constantly as it thickens. Stir in the egg yolk and the sweetener, remove from heat, and let cool.

To cook in microwave:

In a large bowl combine the cocoa powder, instant coffee, cornstarch, and milk until smooth. Microwave on high, uncovered, for 3 minutes, stir, then microwave 3 more minutes. Fold the beaten egg yolk into the hot mocha mixture, and microwave 2 more minutes. Remove from the microwave, stir in the sweetener, then let cool.

3. In a separate bowl beat the egg whites until soft peaks form, add the cream of tartar, then beat until stiff. Carefully fold the egg whites into the chocolate mixture, mixing just until no whites show. Spoon the mousse into 8 parfait glasses, and chill until serving. This will keep in the refrigerator for several days, tightly covered.

Yield: Makes 8 ½-cup servings

Each serving has approximately 52 calories, 3.6 g. protein, 1.2 g. total fat (0.6 g. unsaturated fat, 0.5 g. saturated fat), 7.3 g. carbohydrates, 27 mg. cholesterol, 0.6 g. fiber, 46 mg. sodium, 84 mg. calcium. Exchanges per serving: ¼ fat, ¼ milk, ¼ starch.

Fruity Couscous Pudding

This exotic relative of rice pudding is sweet and spongy, with chewy bits of dried fruit, and very easy to make.

¾ cup couscous	2 tablespoons raisins
3¼ cups skim milk	2 tablespoons chopped dates
3 tablespoons brown sugar	⅛ teaspoon nutmeg
2 tablespoons orange juice concentrate	

1. Combine all the ingredients in a heavy 2½-quart pot, and cook over low heat, covered, for 10 minutes.

Yield: Makes 8 ⅓-cup servings

Each serving has approximately 121 calories, 5.1 g. protein, 0.2 g. total fat (0.1 g. unsaturated fat, 0.1 g. saturated fat), 25 g. carbohydrates, 1.6 mg. cholesterol, 0.4 g. fiber, 56 mg. sodium, 131 mg. calcium. Exchanges per serving: ¾ fruit, ½ milk, ½ starch.

Chocolate-Covered Bananas

Cool and creamy bananas encased in crunchy cocoa for low-calorie freezer-ready treats.

3 tablespoons unsweetened cocoa powder	¼ cup skim milk
2 packets non-nutritive sweetener	2 firm bananas, each cut in half
	4 6-inch bamboo skewers

1. In a 2-cup glass measuring cup combine the cocoa, sweetener, and milk, and stir until smooth.

2. Carefully insert a bamboo skewer lengthwise into a banana half, then lower it into the chocolate mixture to coat it. Remove the banana from the bowl and lay it on a small tray lined with wax paper. Repeat for the remaining 3 banana halves, then freeze them for 45 minutes. Reserve the remaining chocolate mixture.

3. Remove the bananas from the freezer. Redip each banana in the chocolate mixture. Return to the tray and refreeze for 45 minutes. Set the remaining chocolate mixture aside.

4. Remove the bananas from the freezer, and redip in the chocolate mixture for the third time, then freeze for another 45 minutes.

5. Wrap each chocolate-covered banana tightly in plastic or foil, and store in the freezer.

Yield: Serves 4

Each serving has approximately 68 calories, 1.8 g. protein, 1 g. total fat (0.4 g. unsaturated fat, 0.6 g. saturated fat), 16 g. carbohydrates, 0.3 mg. cholesterol, 2.4 g. fiber, 9.2 mg. sodium, 28 mg. calcium. Exchanges per serving: 1 fruit, ¼ starch.

Raspberry Creme

Cool, fruity, and creamy, with a slight tang from the yogurt.

⅓ cup cold water
1 envelope (⅓ ounce) unsweetened gelatin
1½ cups fresh raspberries or 12
   ounces frozen raspberries,
   defrosted

1 cup plain non-fat yogurt
4 packets non-nutritive
   sweetener

1. Put the cold water in a small saucepan, and sprinkle the gelatin on top. Let sit for 3 minutes to absorb the gelatin. Heat the gelatin mixture over low heat until the gelatin granules dissolve, frequently scraping the sides of the pan.

2. Set ½ cup of the raspberries aside. In a blender or food processor puree the remaining raspberries, yogurt, and sweetener until smooth. Add the gelatin and puree for 10 seconds, then stir in the remaining raspberries with a spoon.

3. Spoon the raspberry creme into four parfait glasses and refrigerate until set.

Yield: Serves 4

Each ¾-cup serving has approximately 65 calories, 5.2 g. protein, 0.4 g. total fat (0.2 g. unsaturated fat, 0.1 g. saturated fat), 10.7 g. carbohydrates, 1 mg. cholesterol, 3.1 g. fiber, 45 mg. sodium, 123 mg. calcium.
Exchanges per serving: ⅔ fruit, ¼ milk.

Frozen Strawberry Sorbet

Icy, sweet, and quick to whip up, it's ready to eat or freeze — a case of having your sorbet and eating it, too.

4 cups whole unsweetened
  frozen strawberries
  (20-ounce bag)
4 tablespoons vanilla non-fat
  yogurt

2 packets non-nutritive
  sweetener
4 sprigs of mint

1. Puree the frozen strawberries in food processor until crumbly. Let rest for 30 seconds.

2. Add the yogurt and sweetener, and puree until smooth, scraping down the sides of the food processor. Transfer to a 1-quart plastic container, cover, and freeze.

3. Before serving, let sit at room temperature for 5 minutes, and garnish each serving with a sprig of mint.

Yield: Makes 4 ¾-cup servings
Each serving has approximately 60 calories, 1.4 g. protein, 0.2 g. total fat (0.1 g. unsaturated fat, 0 g. saturated fat), 14.7 g. carbohydrates, 0.3 mg. cholesterol, 3.9 g. fiber, 13.8 mg. sodium, 51 mg. calcium. Exchanges per serving: 1 fruit.

Mango Sorbet

Smooth, cool, and entirely fresh fruit. You can make it in an ice cream freezer, but it's just as good this way.

3 cups cubed ripe mango (about
  5 or 6 mangoes)
1 ripe banana

1 tablespoon lime juice
½ teaspoon grated lime peel

1. Puree the mango and banana in a food processor. Transfer to a small metal bowl. Stir in the lime juice and lime peel, and cover tightly with plastic wrap.

2. Freeze until firm, about 2 hours.

3. Remove from the freezer, let soften slightly, and beat until

smooth in a food processor. Transfer to a metal bowl and refreeze for 1½ hours.

4. Remove from the freezer, let soften slightly, and beat until smooth in a food processor. Serve.

Yield: Makes 6 ½-cup servings

Each serving has approximately 73 calories, 0.6 g. protein, 0.3 g. total fat (0.2 g. unsaturated fat, 0.1 g. saturated fat), 18.7 g. carbohydrates, 0 mg. cholesterol, 3.3 g. fiber, 1.7 mg. sodium, 9.9 mg. calcium. Exchanges per serving: 1¼ fruit.

Fruity Frozen Yogurt Pops

Creamy, cold, and intensely fruity. Beats store-bought pops hands down.

⅔ **cup plain non-fat yogurt**	2 **packets non-nutritive**
⅔ **cup fresh strawberries**	**sweetener**

1. Combine all the ingredients in a food processor or blender until the berries are pureed.

2. Pour the mixture into 5-ounce paper cups, and place in freezer. When the pops are partially frozen (about 1½ hours), insert a popsicle stick in the center of each cup, and continue freezing for another 1½ hours.

Or use small plastic popsicle molds, available in kitchen supply stores with instructions for freezing.

Yield: Makes 4 popsicles

Each serving has approximately 29 calories, 2.3 g. protein, 0.15 g. total fat (0.07 g. unsaturated fat, 0.05 g. saturated fat), 4.9 g. carbohydrates, 0.7 mg. cholesterol, 0.6 g. fiber, 28 mg. sodium, 78 mg. calcium. Exchanges per serving: ½ fruit.

Orange Cream Pops

A no-fat, low-calorie version of a childhood favorite.

¾ cup plain non-fat yogurt
¼ cup orange juice concentrate
 2 packets non-nutritive
   sweetener (optional)

1. In a bowl combine the yogurt and orange juice concentrate. Taste for sweetness, and add non-nutritive sweetener to your liking.

2. Pour the mixture into 4 plastic popsicle molds or 5-ounce paper cups, insert popsicle sticks, and freeze for 2 hours.

Yield: Makes 4 ½-cup pops

Each serving has approximately 51 calories, 2.5 g. protein, 0.1 g. total fat (0 g. unsaturated fat, 0.1 g. saturated fat), 10.3 g. carbohydrates, 0.8 mg. cholesterol, 0.2 g. fiber, 31 mg. sodium, 90 mg. calcium. Exchanges per serving: ½ fruit, ¼ milk.

Beverages

Strawberry Banana Shake
Frozen Eggnog
Brandy Pumpkin Milk Shake
Minty Hot Chocolate
Cinnamon Mocha Cocoa
Chocolate Mint Milk Shake
Mocha Shake
Creamy Coconut Shake

Piña Colada
Iced Espresso
Coffee-Flavored Root Beer
  Float
Creamy Cranberry-Orange
  Smoothie
Cantaloupe Lime Cooler
Spiced Apple Smoothie
Peach Milk Shake

Strawberry Banana Shake

Cool and creamy, with a sweet fruity taste.

⅔ cup orange juice
⅔ cup non-fat plain yogurt
⅔ cup fresh strawberries
½ banana

6 ice cubes
2 packets non-nutritive
   sweetener, to taste

1. Combine all the ingredients in a blender or food processor and puree for 30 seconds, or until smooth and creamy.

Yield: Makes 4 ¾-cup servings
Each serving has approximately 59 calories, 2.4 g. protein, 0.3 g. total fat (0.1 g. unsaturated fat, 0.1 g. saturated fat), 12.5 g. carbohydrates, 0.7 mg. cholesterol, 1 g. fiber, 27 mg. sodium, 83 mg. calcium. Exchanges per serving: ⅔ fruit, ¼ milk.

Frozen Eggnog

Tastes like the real thing in a frothy-shake version.

¼ cup liquid cholesterol-free egg
   replacement, like Egg Beaters
½ cup vanilla ice milk
1 cup skim milk

¼ teaspoon rum extract
4 ice cubes
ground nutmeg, for garnish

1. Combine all the ingredients except the nutmeg in a blender, and puree for 30 seconds, until smooth. Pour into tall glasses and sprinkle with a dash of nutmeg.

Yield: Makes 3 ¾-cup servings
Each serving has approximately 77 calories, 6.2 g. protein, 1.8 g. total fat (0.9 g. unsaturated fat, 0.8 g. saturated fat), 8.9 g. carbohydrates, 4.6 mg. cholesterol, 0 g. fiber, 96.5 mg. sodium, 141 mg. calcium. Exchanges per serving: ⅓ fat, ⅓ milk, ⅓ starch.

Brandy Pumpkin Milk Shake

Thick and rich shake, and flavored with nutmeg and a hint of brandy.

½ cup vanilla ice milk	⅛ teaspoon nutmeg
½ cup canned pumpkin puree	¼ teaspoon brandy extract
1 cup skim milk	¼ cup crushed ice or 4 ice cubes

1. Combine all the ingredients in a blender, and puree for 30 seconds, until smooth.

Yield: Makes 3 ¾-cup servings

Each serving has approximately 68 calories, 4 g. protein, 1.2 g. total fat (0.4 g. unsaturated fat, 0.7 g. saturated fat), 11 g. carbohydrates, 4.3 mg. cholesterol, 0.7 g. fiber, 60 mg. sodium, 136 mg. calcium. Exchanges per serving: ¼ fat, ⅓ milk, ⅓ starch.

Minty Hot Chocolate

¾ cup skim milk	1 packet non-nutritive sweetener
1 tablespoon unsweetened cocoa powder	2 drops mint extract

1. Combine all the ingredients well with a whisk, or whiz in a blender or food processor until free of lumps.

2. Pour the mixture into a small saucepan and heat over low heat until warm, or into a microwave-safe mug, and cook on high for 2 minutes.

Yield: Makes 1 ¾-cup serving

Each serving has approximately 74 calories, 6.8 g. protein, 1.4 g. total fat (0.6 g. unsaturated fat, 0.8 g. saturated fat), 10.8 g. carbohydrates, 2.8 mg. cholesterol, 1.6 g. fiber, 88.6 mg. sodium, 218 mg. calcium. Exchanges per serving: 1 milk.

Cinnamon Mocha Cocoa

Chocolate and cinnamon spice a warm coffee drink.

¾ cup skim milk
1 tablespoon unsweetened cocoa powder

⅛ teaspoon cinnamon
2 teaspoons instant coffee
1 packet non-nutritive sweetener

1. Combine all the ingredients in a microwave-safe mug, and microwave on high for 2 minutes, or heat in a saucepan over very low heat until warm.

Yield: Makes 1 ¾-cup serving
Each serving has approximately 78 calories, 6.7 g. protein, 1.3 g. total fat (0.5 g. unsaturated fat, 0.8 g. saturated fat), 12. g. carbohydrates, 2.8 mg. cholesterol, 1.7 g. fiber, 88.6 mg. sodium, 221 mg. calcium. Exchanges per serving: 1 milk.

Chocolate Mint Milk Shake

Rich, frothy, and as chocolate as a low-cal shake can get.

¼ cup chocolate ice milk
½ cup non-fat milk
⅛ teaspoon mint extract

1. Whip the ingredients in a blender or food processor.

Yield: Makes 1 ¾-cup serving
Each serving has approximately 89 calories, 5.5 g. protein, 1.6 g. total fat (0.5 g. unsaturated fat, 1 g. saturated fat), 13 g. carbohydrates, 6.5 mg. cholesterol, 0 g. fiber, 89 mg. sodium, 195 mg. calcium. Exchanges per serving: ¼ fat, ½ milk, ½ starch.

Mocha Shake

A frothy and sweet coffee-chocolate-flavored shake with a hint of cinnamon.

¾ cup skim milk	2 ice cubes
2 teaspoons instant coffee powder	2 packets non-nutritive sweetener
1 teaspoon chocolate extract	dash cinnamon

1. Combine the milk, instant coffee powder, chocolate extract, ice cubes, and sweetener in a blender, and blend for 10 seconds.

2. Pour into a tall glass and sprinkle with a dash of cinnamon.

Yield: Makes 1 10-ounce serving

Each serving has approximately 68 calories, 5.8 g. protein, 0.3 g. total fat (0.1 g. unsaturated fat, 0.2 g. saturated fat), 10.3 g. carbohydrates, 2.8 mg. cholesterol, 0 g. fiber, 87.5 mg. sodium, 210 mg. calcium. Exchanges per serving: ¾ milk.

Creamy Coconut Shake

¾ cup skim milk	2 packets non-nutritive sweetener
½ teaspoon coconut extract	1 sprig of mint
½ teaspoon vanilla extract	
2 ice cubes	

1. Combine the milk, coconut and vanilla extracts, ice cubes, and sweetener in a blender, and blend for 10 seconds.

2. Pour into a tall glass and garnish with a sprig of mint.

Yield: Makes 1 10-ounce serving

Each serving has approximately 68 calories, 5.8 g. protein, 0.3 g. total fat (0.1 g. unsaturated fat, 0.2 g. saturated fat), 10.3 g. carbohydrates, 2.8 mg. cholesterol, 0 g. fiber, 87.5 mg. sodium, 210 mg. calcium. Exchanges per serving: ¾ milk.

Piña Colada

Cool, creamy, and filling.

¾ cup unsweetened crushed
  pineapple
¾ cup plain non-fat yogurt
½ cup crushed ice or ¾ cup ice
  cubes

½ teaspoon coconut extract
1 packet non-nutritive sweetener
2 sprigs fresh mint

1. Combine all the ingredients in a blender, and puree until smooth. Garnish with mint.

Yield: Makes 2 1-cup servings
Each serving has approximately 93 calories, 4.5 g. protein, 0.2 g. total fat (0.1 g. unsaturated fat, 0.1 g. saturated fat), 19 g. carbohydrates, 2 mg. cholesterol, 0.8 g. fiber, 61 mg. sodium, 181 mg. calcium.
Exchanges per serving: ¾ fruit, ½ milk.

Iced Espresso

The evaporated skim milk, rather than plain skim milk, makes this iced coffee surprisingly creamy and rich.

¾ cup brewed espresso coffee
3 ounces evaporated skim milk
1 packet non-nutritive sweetener

1. Combine all the ingredients, stir, and pour over ice.

Yield: Makes 1 9-ounce serving
Each serving has approximately 72 calories, 6.4 g. protein, 0.2 g. total fat (0 g. unsaturated fat, 0.1 g. saturated fat), 11.4 g. carbohydrates, 3.3 mg. cholesterol, 0 g. fiber, 102 mg. sodium, 249 mg. calcium.
Exchanges per serving: ⅔ milk.

Coffee-Flavored Root Beer Float

Cold, refreshing root beer treat with a new twist.

¾ **cup ice cubes**
1 **cup diet root beer**
¼ **cup vanilla ice milk, slightly**
  softened
1 **teaspoon instant coffee**

1. Combine the ice and root beer in a 12-ounce glass.
2. Put the ice milk in a bowl or glass measuring cup, stir in the instant coffee, and add this to the root beer.

Yield: Makes 1 12-ounce serving
Each serving has approximately 49 calories, 1.3 g. protein, 1.4 g. total fat (0.5 g. unsaturated fat, 0.9 g. saturated fat), 8 g. carbohydrates, 4.5 mg. cholesterol, 0 g. fiber, 47 mg. sodium, 55 mg. calcium. Exchanges per serving: ⅓ fat, ⅓ starch.

Creamy Cranberry-Orange Smoothie

Tart cranberry, sweet orange, and creamy yogurt make a cooling drink.

¾ **cup low-calorie cranberry juice**   ¼ **teaspoon orange extract**
½ **cup orange juice**   ½ **cup ice cubes**
¼ **cup plain non-fat yogurt**   2 **orange slices, for garnish**

1. Puree all the ingredients in a blender or food processor. Garnish with an orange slice and serve.

Yield: Makes 2 1-cup servings
Each serving has approximately 59 calories, 1.8 g. protein, 0.2 g. total fat (0.1 g. unsaturated fat, 0.1 g. saturated fat), 12.8 g. carbohydrates, 0.5 mg. cholesterol, 0.2 g. fiber, 25 mg. sodium, 63 mg. calcium. Exchanges per serving: ⅔ fruit, ⅛ milk.

Cantaloupe Lime Cooler

Fruity and cool, with the tang of lime.

¼ small cantaloupe, seeded and
   cubed
⅓ cup plain non-fat yogurt
1 tablespoon lime juice

½ cup ice cubes
1 packet non-nutritive sweetener
⅛ teaspoon grated lime peel

1. Puree all the ingredients together in a blender or food processor until smooth. Garnish with grated lime peel.

Yield: Makes 1 10-ounce serving

Each serving has approximately 92 calories, 4.9 g. protein, 0.5 g. total fat (0.2 g. unsaturated fat, 0.2 g. saturated fat), 19 g. carbohydrates, 1.3 mg. cholesterol, 1.4 g. fiber, 65 mg. sodium, 165 mg. calcium. Exchanges per serving: 1 fruit, ⅓ milk.

Spiced Apple Smoothie

Sweet apple shake with earthy spices.

1 Granny Smith apple, peeled
   and sliced
½ cup plain non-fat yogurt
1 teaspoon vanilla extract
⅓ cup skim milk

2 packets non-nutritive
   sweetener
½ teaspoon cinnamon
⅛ teaspoon nutmeg
½ cup ice cubes

1. Combine all the ingredients except the ice cubes in a blender or food processor, and puree until smooth. Add the ice cubes, and puree until ice is crushed.

Yield: Makes 2 1-cup servings

Each serving has approximately 83 calories, 4.2 g. protein, 0.4 g. total fat (0.2 g. unsaturated fat, 0.2 g. saturated fat), 17 g. carbohydrates, 1.7 mg. cholesterol, 1.5 g. fiber, 61 mg. sodium, 172 mg. calcium. Exchanges per serving: ¾ fruit, ½ milk.

Peach Milk Shake

Peachy, smooth, and thick.

½ cup vanilla ice milk
1 can (8-ounce) sugar-free peach halves

½ cup skim milk
¼ cup crushed ice or 4 ice cubes

1. Combine all the ingredients in a blender, and puree for 30 seconds, until smooth.

Yield: Makes 3 ¾-cup servings

Each serving has approximately 78 calories, 3 g. protein, 1 g. total fat (0.3 g. unsaturated fat, 0.6 g. saturated fat), 15.6 g. carbohydrates, 4 mg. cholesterol, 0.9 g. fiber, 41 mg. sodium, 84.6 mg. calcium. Exchanges per serving: ¼ fat, ½ fruit, ¼ milk, ⅓ starch.

IV. Menu Planner

HERE are three fourteen-day meal plans based on the tasty high-flavor, high-texture recipes in this book. The first provides 1300 calories a day; the second, 1500 calories a day; and the third, 2000 calories a day. Choose the one that suits your present needs.

Each menu plan provides a nutritionally sound, low-fat, low-cholesterol diet high in complex carbohydrates with moderate amounts of protein. If you are not familiar with the current high-carbohydrate recommendations, you may be surprised at the amounts of such foods as bread, pasta, rice, and, yes, popcorn that are part of the meal plans.

You can also supplement your meals and snacks with unlimited quantities of the following vegetables and drinks: lettuce, celery, chicory, cucumber, parsley, radishes, watercress, club soda, seltzer, mineral water, diet sodas, sugar-free tonic, decaffeinated coffee and tea, and herb teas.

For those of you who work with food exchanges, the meal plans conform to the exchange system used by the American Diabetic Association and American Dietetic Association that divides all approved foods into six groups — starches, low-fat meats, vegetables, fruits, low-fat milks, and fats. Each portion of food is given its exchange value based on its calories and nutritional content. The 1300-calorie day provides 8 starches, 3 low-fat meats, 3 vegetables, 2 fruits, 2 low-fat milks, and 3 fats. The 1500-calorie day provides 9 starches, 3 low-fat meats, 6 vegetables, 2 fruits, 2 low-fat milks, and 4 fats. The 2000-calorie day provides 12 starches, 4 low-fat meats, 6 vegetables, 3 fruits, 3 low-fat milks, and 5 fats.

1300 Calories — Day 1

Breakfast:

- 1 cup non-fat yogurt
- 1¼ cup fresh strawberries
- 1 slice whole wheat toast
- 1 teaspoon margarine

Snack:

- 2 **Whole Wheat Blueberry Muffins**

Lunch:

- 1 serving **Italian Antipasto Salad**
- ¾ cup **Tomato Clam Soup**
- 4 **Herbed Whole Wheat Bread Sticks**

Snack:

- 10 ounces **Creamy Coconut Shake**

Dinner:

- 1 serving **Fish Fillets with Red Pepper Glaze**
- ⅔ cup **Wild and Brown Rice**
- ½ cup steamed yellow squash
- 1 **Rye Dinner Roll**
- 1 teaspoon margarine
- 1 serving **Frozen Strawberry Sorbet**

1300 Calories — Day 2

Breakfast:

- 1 whole wheat English muffin
- 1 teaspoon margarine
- ½ grapefruit

Snack:

- ¾ cup **Strawberry Banana Shake**

Lunch:

- 1 serving **Poached Fish with Julienne Vegetables**
- 1 cup **Cold Creamy Cucumber Soup**

Snack:

- 3 cups **Parmesan Popcorn**

Dinner:

- 1 serving **Spicy Italian "Meatballs" with Spaghetti**
- 1 small whole wheat roll
- 1 teaspoon margarine
- 1 cup cooked broccoli
- 1 small salad
- 1 tablespoon **Fresh Herb Vinaigrette**
- 1 piece **Chocolate Cake**
- 1 cup skim milk

1300 Calories — Day 3

Breakfast:

- 1 toasted bagel
- 2 tablespoons **Smoked Salmon Spread**
- ½ cup non-fat yogurt
- ½ banana, sliced

Snack:

- 1 **Orange Cream Pop**

Lunch:

- 1 cup **Fish Chowder**
- 2 servings **Wild Rice Frittata**
- ¾ cup **Creamy Cucumber and Onions**

Snack:

- ¾ cup **Peach Milk Shake**

Dinner:

- 1 cup **Cajun Jambalaya Rice**
- 1 serving **Hot and Daring Zucchini Creole**
- 1 **Sweet Potato Biscuit**
- 1 teaspoon margarine
- 1 slice **Blueberry Cream Cheese Pie**

1300 Calories — Day 4

Breakfast:

- 2 **Strawberry Crepes**
- ¾ cup **Cinnamon Mocha Cocoa**

Snack:

- 1 **Applesauce Walnut Bran Muffin**
- ½ teaspoon margarine

Lunch:

- 1½ cups **Pasta Fagioli**
- 1 whole wheat roll
- 1 teaspoon margarine

Snack:

- 1 cup **Spiced Apple Smoothie**

Dinner:

- 1 serving **Baked Tuna Niçoise**
- 1 serving **Herbed Whole New Potatoes**
- 6 stalks steamed asparagus
- ½ teaspoon margarine
- 1 piece **Key Lime Pie**

1300 Calories — Day 5

Breakfast:

- ¾ cup cooked oatmeal
- ¾ cup skim milk
- 1 tablespoon raisins

Snack:

- ¾ cup **Frozen Eggnog**

Lunch:

- 1 **Chicken Enchilada**
- ⅔ cup **Mexican Pasta Salad**
- 8 **Homemade Tortilla Chips**

Snack:

- 2 small tangerines

Dinner:

- 1 serving **Lamb Stew**
- ⅔ cup **Lemon Couscous**
- ½ cup steamed zucchini
- 1 piece **Applesauce Cake**
- 1 cup skim milk

1300 Calories — Day 6

Breakfast:

- 1 **Baked Apple with Raspberries and Cognac**
- ½ whole wheat English muffin
- 1 teaspoon margarine

Snack:

- ¾ cup non-fat yogurt
- ¾ cup cubed fresh honeydew melon

Lunch:

- 2 cups **Oriental Vegetable Stir-Fry**
- ⅔ cup cooked brown rice

Snack:

- 3 **Bagel Chips**
- 2 tablespoons **Creamy Herb Dip**

Dinner:

- 1 serving **Chicken Paprikash**
- 1½ ounces dried wide noodles, cooked
- 1 teaspoon margarine
- 1 serving **Sweet and Sour Red Cabbage**

Snack:

- 2 **Apricot Oat Bran Cookies**
- ¾ cup skim milk

1300 Calories — Day 7

Breakfast:

1½ ounces unsweetened cereal
½ cup skim milk
½ cup fresh strawberries

Snack:

1 apple

Lunch:

¾ cup **Herbed Tomato Soup**
1¾ cups **Penne with Basil and Sweet Peppers**

Snack:

1½ ounces unsalted pretzels

Dinner:

1 serving **Bluefish with Spicy Salsa**
2 **Jalapeño Corn Biscuits**
½ teaspoon margarine
1 serving **Butternut Squash with Maple Glaze**
1 serving **Figs in a Chocolate Pool**
¾ cup skim milk

1300 Calories — Day 8

Breakfast:

2 **Blintzes**
2 tablespoons non-fat yogurt
¾ cup blueberries

Snack:

1 **Cinnamon Bun**
½ teaspoon margarine

Lunch:

¾ cup **Succotash Soup**
1 serving **Broccoli-Stuffed Potato**

Snack:

1¼ cups watermelon cubes

Dinner:

1 serving **Pork Tenderloin with Chutney Glaze**
¾ cup baked acorn squash
½ teaspoon margarine
1 serving **Sautéed Radicchio and Watercress**
1 **Butterscotch Square**
¾ cup skim milk

1300 Calories — Day 9

Breakfast:

- ½ grapefruit
- 2 **Corn Pancakes**
- 1 teaspoon margarine
- 2 tablespoons low-calorie syrup

Snack:

- 2 small plums

Lunch:

- ¾ cup **Creamy Orange Carrot Soup**
- 1 serving **White Bean Salad with Tomato Basil Vinaigrette**
- 1 whole wheat roll
- ½ teaspoon margarine

Snack:

- ¾ cup **Brandy Pumpkin Milk Shake**

Dinner:

- 3 ounces **Tandoori Chicken**
- 1 serving **Spinach Sag Paneer**
- ⅔ cup cooked brown rice

Snack:

- ½ cup **Mocha Mousse**
- ¾ cup skim milk

1300 Calories — Day 10

Breakfast:

- 2 slices **Pumpkin Bread**
- 1 teaspoon margarine
- ½ cup low-fat (1%) cottage cheese

Snack:

- ¾ cup cubed fresh pineapple

Lunch:

- 2 skewers **Beef Teriyaki**
- ½ cup brown rice
- ¾ cup **Marinated Radishes**

Snack:

- ¾ cup **Minty Hot Chocolate**
- 2 **Poppy Seed Cookies with Raspberry Jam**

Dinner:

- 1 serving **Angel Hair with Scallops and Crabmeat**
- 1 serving **Broccoli with Anchovies**
- 1 whole wheat roll
- 1 teaspoon margarine
- ¾ cup **Raspberry Creme**
- ½ cup skim milk

1300 Calories — Day 11

Breakfast:

- ¾ cup cooked cereal
- ½ cup skim milk
- 1 small apple

Snack:

- 1 slice **Cranberry Nut Bread**
- ½ cup skim milk

Lunch:

- ¾ cup **Sweet Potato Soup**
- 1 serving **Fettuccine with Mushroom Stroganoff**

Snack:

- 2 cups **Caramel Popcorn**

Dinner:

- 1 serving **Chicken with Tarragon Sauce**
- ½ baked potato
- 1 teaspoon margarine
- ½ cup steamed green beans
- 1 serving **Peach Crisp**
- ½ cup skim milk

1300 Calories — Day 12

Breakfast:

- 1 serving **Poached Pears in Cranberry Glaze**
- ¾ cup cooked oatmeal
- 1 teaspoon margarine
- ½ cup skim milk

Snack:

- ¾ cup **Mocha Shake**

Lunch:

- 1 cup **Six-Vegetable Chowder**
- 2 **Poppy Seed Biscuits**
- 1 teaspoon margarine

Snack:

- 1 serving **Coffee-Flavored Root Beer Float**

Dinner:

- 3 ounces **Veal Loaf**
- 1 serving **Peppery Mushroom Sauce**
- 1 cup steamed broccoli
- 1 cup **Mashed Potatoes**
- 1 teaspoon margarine
- 1 **Chocolate-Covered Banana**
- ½ cup skim milk

1300 Calories — Day 13

Breakfast:

- 2 **Blueberry Oatmeal Pancakes**
- 2 tablespoons low-calorie syrup
- ⅓ cantaloupe

Snack:

- ¾ cup **Chocolate Mint Milk Shake**

Lunch:

- 1 cup **Vegetable Barley Soup**
- 1 cup **Black Bean Confetti Salad**
- ½ baked potato
- ½ teaspoon margarine

Snack:

- ⅓ cup **Fruity Couscous Pudding**

Dinner:

- 1 **Three-Herb Crab Cake**
- 2 tablespoons **Tartar Sauce**
- 1 serving **Creamy Country Beets**
- 1 serving **Almost French-Fried Potatoes**
- 1 serving **Pumpkin Pie**
- 1 cup skim milk

1300 Calories — Day 14

Breakfast:

- 3-egg-white omelet
- ⅓ cup **Spicy Salsa**
- 1 **Homemade Flour Tortilla with Scallions**

Snack:

- 1 **Banana Walnut Muffin**
- ½ cup skim milk

Lunch:

- 1 serving **Salmon-Stuffed Baked Potato**
- 1½ cups **Caesar Salad**

Snack:

- 8 ounces **Piña Colada**

Dinner:

- ¾ cup **Cream of Broccoli Soup**
- 1 serving **Turkey-Stuffed Peppers**
- 2 5-inch ears of corn
- 1 teaspoon margarine
- 1 slice **Strawberry Rhubarb Pie**

1500 Calories—Day 1

Breakfast:

1   cup non-fat yogurt
1¼ cup fresh strawberries
1   slice whole wheat toast
1   teaspoon margarine

Snack:

2   **Whole Wheat Blueberry Muffins**
1   teaspoon margarine
9   ounces **Iced Espresso**

Lunch:

1   serving **Italian Antipasto Salad**
¾   cup **Tomato Clam Soup**
4   **Herbed Whole Wheat Bread Sticks**

Snack:

1   medium orange

Dinner:

1   serving **Fish Fillets with Red Pepper Glaze**
⅔   cup **Wild and Brown Rice**
1   **Rye Dinner Roll**
1   teaspoon margarine
1   cup steamed yellow squash
2   pieces **Apple Strudel**
½   cup skim milk

1500 Calories—Day 2

Breakfast:

1   whole wheat English muffin
1   teaspoon margarine
½   grapefruit

Snack:

¾   cup **Strawberry Banana Shake**

Lunch:

1   serving **Poached Fish with Julienne Vegetables**
1   cup **Cold Creamy Cucumber Soup**
1   whole wheat roll
1   teaspoon margarine

Snack:

5   cups **Parmesan Popcorn**

Dinner:

1   serving **Spicy Italian "Meatballs" with Spaghetti**
1   small whole wheat roll
1   teaspoon margarine
1   cup cooked broccoli
1   small salad
1   tablespoon **Fresh Herb Vinaigrette**
1   piece **Chocolate Cake**
¾   cup skim milk

1500 Calories — Day 3

Breakfast:

- 1 toasted bagel
- 2 tablespoons **Smoked Salmon Spread**
- ½ cup non-fat yogurt
- ½ banana, sliced

Snack:

- 1 **Orange Cream Pop**

Lunch:

- 1 cup **Fish Chowder**
- 2 servings **Wild Rice Frittata**
- ¾ cup **Creamy Cucumber and Onions**

Snack:

- ¾ cup **Peach Milk Shake**

Dinner:

- 1½ cups **Cajun Jambalaya Rice**
- 1 serving **Hot and Daring Zucchini Creole**
- ½ cup steamed collard greens
- 1 **Sweet Potato Biscuit**
- 1 teaspoon margarine
- 1 slice **Blueberry Cream Cheese Pie**

1500 Calories — Day 4

Breakfast:

- 2 **Strawberry Crepes**
- ¾ cup **Cinnamon Mocha Cocoa**

Snack:

- 1 **Applesauce Walnut Bran Muffin**
- 1 teaspoon margarine

Lunch:

- 1½ cups **Pasta Fagioli**
- 1 whole wheat roll
- 1 teaspoon margarine
- ½ cup steamed green beans

Snack:

- 1 cup **Spiced Apple Smoothie**

Dinner:

- 1 serving **Baked Tuna Niçoise**
- 2 servings **Herbed Whole New Potatoes**
- 6 stalks steamed asparagus
- ½ teaspoon margarine
- 1 piece **Key Lime Pie**
- ½ cup skim milk

1500 Calories—Day 5

Breakfast:

¾ cup cooked oatmeal
¾ cup skim milk
1 tablespoon raisins
1 slice whole wheat toast
1 teaspoon margarine

Snack:

¾ cup **Frozen Eggnog**

Lunch:

1 **Chicken Enchilada**
1 cup **Mexican Pasta Salad**
8 **Homemade Tortilla Chips**

Snack:

2 small tangerines

Dinner:

1 serving **Lamb Stew**
⅔ cup **Lemon Couscous**
1 cup steamed zucchini
1 piece **Applesauce Cake**
1 cup skim milk

1500 Calories—Day 6

Breakfast:

1 **Baked Apple with Rasp-
    berries and Cognac**
1 whole wheat English muffin
1 teaspoon margarine

Snack:

¾ cup non-fat yogurt
6 almonds
¾ cup cubed fresh honeydew
    melon

Lunch:

2 cups **Oriental Vegetable
    Stir-Fry**
1 cup cooked brown rice

Snack:

3 **Bagel Chips**
2 tablespoons **Creamy Herb Dip**

Dinner:

1 serving **Chicken Paprikash**
1½ ounces dried wide noodles,
    cooked
1 teaspoon margarine
1 serving **Sweet and Sour Red
    Cabbage**
2 **Apricot Oat Bran Cookies**
¾ cup skim milk

1500 Calories — Day 7

Breakfast:

1½ ounces unsweetened cereal
½ cup skim milk
½ cup fresh strawberries

Snack:

1 apple

Lunch:

¾ cup **Herbed Tomato Soup**
1¾ cups **Penne with Basil and Sweet Peppers**
2 slices **Baked Eggplant with Pesto**

Snack:

1½ ounces pretzels

Dinner:

1 serving **Bluefish with Spicy Salsa**
2 **Jalapeño Corn Biscuits**
1 teaspoon margarine
1 serving **Butternut Squash with Maple Glaze**
1 serving **Figs in a Chocolate Pool**
1 cup skim milk

1500 Calories — Day 8

Breakfast:

2 **Blintzes**
2 tablespoons non-fat yogurt
¾ cup blueberries

Snack:

1 **Cinnamon Bun**
1 teaspoon margarine

Lunch:

¾ cup **Succotash Soup**
1 serving **Broccoli-Stuffed Potato**

Snack:

1¼ cups watermelon cubes

Dinner:

1 serving **Pork Tenderloin with Chutney Glaze**
1½ cups baked acorn squash
1 teaspoon margarine
1 serving **Sautéed Radicchio and Watercress**
1 cup steamed cauliflower
1 **Butterscotch Square**
1 cup skim milk

1500 Calories — Day 9

Breakfast:

½ grapefruit
3 **Corn Pancakes**
1 teaspoon margarine
2 tablespoons low-calorie syrup

Snack:

2 small plums

Lunch:

¾ cup **Creamy Orange Carrot Soup**
1 serving **White Bean Salad with Tomato Basil Vinaigrette**
1 whole wheat roll
1 teaspoon margarine

Snack:

¾ cup **Brandy Pumpkin Milk Shake**

Dinner:

3 ounces **Tandoori Chicken**
1 serving **Spinach Sag Paneer**
1 serving **Indian Curried Vegetables**
¾ cup cooked brown rice
½ cup **Mocha Mousse**
¾ cup skim milk

1500 Calories — Day 10

Breakfast:

2 slices **Pumpkin Bread**
1 teaspoon margarine
2 teaspoons reduced-sugar jam
½ cup low-fat (1%) cottage cheese

Snack:

¾ cup cubed fresh pineapple
¾ cup non-fat yogurt

Lunch:

2 skewers **Beef Teriyaki**
½ cup brown rice
¾ cup **Marinated Radishes**

Snack:

¾ cup **Minty Hot Chocolate**
4 **Poppy Seed Cookies with Raspberry Jam**

Dinner:

1 serving **Angel Hair with Scallops and Crabmeat**
1 serving **Broccoli with Anchovies**
1 whole wheat roll
1 teaspoon margarine
¾ cup **Raspberry Creme**
½ cup skim milk

1500 Calories — Day 11

Breakfast:

- ¾ cup cooked cereal
- ½ cup skim milk
- 1 small apple

Snack:

- 1 slice **Cranberry Nut Bread**
- ½ cup skim milk

Lunch:

- ¾ cup **Sweet Potato Soup**
- 1 serving **Fettuccine with Mushroom Stroganoff**
- 1 whole wheat roll
- 1 teaspoon margarine

Snack:

- 2 cups **Caramel Popcorn**

Dinner:

- 1 serving **Chicken with Tarragon Sauce**
- 1 baked potato
- 1 teaspoon margarine
- ½ cup steamed green beans
- 1 serving **Peach Crisp**

1500 Calories — Day 12

Breakfast:

- 1 serving **Poached Pears in Cranberry Glaze**
- ¾ cup cooked oatmeal
- 1 teaspoon margarine
- ½ cup skim milk

Snack:

- ¾ cup **Mocha Shake**

Lunch:

- 1 cup **Six-Vegetable Chowder**
- 2 **Poppy Seed Biscuits**
- 1 teaspoon margarine
- 1 small salad
- 2 tablespoons **Sweet Orange Poppy Dressing**

Snack:

- 1 serving **Coffee-Flavored Root Beer Float**
- 1¼ ounces unsalted pretzels

Dinner:

- 3 ounces **Veal Loaf**
- 1 serving **Peppery Mushroom Sauce**
- 1 cup **Mashed Potatoes**
- 1 teaspoon margarine
- 1 serving **Zucchini Parmesan**
- 1 **Chocolate-Covered Banana**
- ½ cup skim milk

1500 Calories—Day 13

Breakfast:

3   **Blueberry Oatmeal Pancakes**
2   tablespoons low-calorie syrup
⅓   cantaloupe

Snack:

¾   cup **Chocolate Mint Milk Shake**

Lunch:

1   cup **Vegetable Barley Soup**
1   cup **Black Bean Confetti Salad**
1   baked potato
1   teaspoon margarine

Snack:

⅓   cup **Fruity Couscous Pudding**

Dinner:

1   **Three-Herb Crab Cake**
2   tablespoons **Tartar Sauce**
1   serving **Creamy Country Beets**
¾   cup steamed brussel sprouts
1   serving **Almost French-Fried Potatoes**
1   serving **Pumpkin Pie**
1   cup skim milk

1500 Calories—Day 14

Breakfast:

3-egg-white omelet
⅓   cup **Spicy Salsa**
1   **Homemade Flour Tortilla with Scallions**

Snack:

1   **Banana Walnut Muffin**
1   teaspoon margarine
½   cup skim milk

Lunch:

2   servings **Salmon-Stuffed Baked Potato**
1½   cups **Caesar Salad**

Snack:

8   ounces **Piña Colada**

Dinner:

¾   cup **Cream of Broccoli Soup**
1   serving **Turkey-Stuffed Peppers**
2   5-inch ears of corn
1   teaspoon margarine
1   slice **Strawberry Rhubarb Pie**

2000 Calories — Day 1

Breakfast:

- 1 cup non-fat yogurt
- 1¼ cup fresh strawberries
- 2 slices whole wheat toast
- 1 teaspoon margarine

Snack:

- 2 **Whole Wheat Blueberry Muffins**
- 1 teaspoon margarine
- 9 ounces **Iced Espresso**

Lunch:

- 1 serving **Italian Antipasto Salad**
- ¾ cup **Tomato Clam Soup**
- 4 **Herbed Whole Wheat Bread Sticks**
- 3 tablespoons **Horseradish Spread**

Snack:

- 1 medium orange
- 1 slice **Pumpkin Bread**

Dinner:

- 1 serving **Fish Fillets with Red Pepper Glaze**
- 1⅓ cups **Wild and Brown Rice**
- 1 **Rye Dinner Roll**
- 1 teaspoon margarine
- 1 cup steamed yellow squash
- 1 small salad
- 2 tablespoons **Cucumber Blue Cheese Dressing**
- 2 pieces **Apple Strudel**
- 1 cup skim milk

2000 Calories — Day 2

Breakfast:

- 1 whole wheat English muffin
- 1 teaspoon margarine
- ½ grapefruit
- 1 cup non-fat yogurt

Snack:

- ¾ cup **Strawberry Banana Shake**
- 1 **Banana Walnut Muffin**
- ½ teaspoon margarine

Lunch:

- 1 serving **Poached Fish with Julienne Vegetables**
- 1 cup **Cold Creamy Cucumber Soup**
- 2 servings **Double Mushroom Sauté with Tarragon**
- 1 whole wheat roll
- 1 teaspoon margarine

Snack:

- 5 cups **Parmesan Popcorn**

Dinner:

- 1½ servings **Spicy Italian "Meatballs" with Spaghetti**
- 1 tablespoon grated Parmesan cheese
- 1 small whole wheat roll
- 1 teaspoon margarine
- 1 cup cooked broccoli
- 1 piece **Chocolate Cake**
- ¾ cup skim milk
- 1 cup fresh raspberries

2000 Calories—Day 3

Breakfast:

- 1 toasted bagel
- 2 tablespoons **Smoked Salmon Spread**
- 1 cup non-fat yogurt
- 1 banana, sliced

Snack:

- 1 **Orange Cream Pop**

Lunch:

- 1 cup **Fish Chowder**
- 2 servings **Wild Rice Frittata**
- ¾ cup **Creamy Cucumber and Onions**
- 1 slice whole wheat bread
- 1 teaspoon margarine

Snack:

- 1 cup **Peach Milk Shake**
- 3 **Bagel Chips**

Dinner:

- 2 cups **Cajun Jambalaya Rice**
- 2 servings **Hot and Daring Zucchini Creole**
- ½ cup steamed collard greens
- 1 **Sweet Potato Biscuit**
- 1 teaspoon margarine
- 1 slice **Blueberry Cream Cheese Pie**
- 1 cup skim milk

2000 Calories—Day 4

Breakfast:

- 3 **Strawberry Crepes**
- ¾ cup **Cinnamon Mocha Cocoa**

Snack:

- 1 **Applesauce Walnut Bran Muffin**
- 1 teaspoon margarine

Lunch:

- 2¼ cups **Pasta Fagioli**
- 1 whole wheat roll
- 1 teaspoon margarine
- ½ cup steamed green beans
- 1 small green salad
- 1 tablespoon **Fresh Herb Vinaigrette**

Snack:

- 1 cup **Spiced Apple Smoothie**

Dinner:

- 1 serving **Baked Tuna Niçoise**
- 2 servings **Herbed Whole New Potatoes**
- 6 stalks steamed asparagus
- 1 **Rye Dinner Roll**
- 1 teaspoon margarine
- 1 piece **Key Lime Pie**
- 1 cup skim milk

2000 Calories — Day 5

Breakfast:

- 1 cup cooked oatmeal
- 1 cup skim milk
- 2 tablespoons raisins
- 1 slice whole wheat toast
- 1 teaspoon margarine

Snack:

- 2 small tangerines

Lunch:

- 1 **Chicken Enchilada**
- 2 ounces plain non-fat yogurt
- ⅛ medium avocado, sliced
- 1 cup **Mexican Pasta Salad**

- 1 serving **Spinach Salad with Smoked Oysters and Orange Vinaigrette Dressing**
- 8 **Homemade Tortilla Chips**

Snack:

- 1½ cups **Frozen Eggnog**
- ¾ ounce unsalted pretzels

Dinner:

- 1 serving **Lamb Stew**
- ⅔ cup **Lemon Couscous**
- 1 cup steamed zucchini
- ½ whole wheat pita bread
- 1 piece **Applesauce Cake**
- 1 cup skim milk

2000 Calories — Day 6

Breakfast:

- 1 **Baked Apple with Raspberries and Cognac**
- 1 whole wheat English muffin
- 1 teaspoon margarine

Snack:

- ¾ cup non-fat yogurt
- 6 almonds
- 1 **Whole Wheat Blueberry Muffin**
- ¾ cup cubed fresh honeydew melon

Lunch:

- 4 cups **Oriental Vegetable Stir-Fry**
- 1 cup cooked brown rice
- ¾ cup fresh blackberries

Snack:

- 6 **Bagel Chips**
- 4 tablespoons **Creamy Herb Dip**

Dinner:

- 1 serving **Chicken Paprikash**
- 2 ounces dried wide noodles, cooked
- 1 teaspoon margarine
- 1 serving **Sweet and Sour Red Cabbage**
- 4 **Apricot Oat Bran Cookies**
- ¾ cup skim milk

2000 Calories — Day 7

Breakfast:

1½ ounces unsweetened cereal
½ cup skim milk
1½ cups fresh strawberries
1 slice rye bread
1 teaspoon margarine

Snack:

1 apple
1 **Poppy Seed Biscuit**

Lunch:

¾ cup **Herbed Tomato Soup**
1¾ cups **Penne with Basil and Sweet Peppers**
4 slices **Baked Eggplant with Pesto**

Snack:

1½ ounces pretzels
¾ cup **Mocha Shake**

Dinner:

1 serving **Bluefish with Spicy Salsa**
2 **Jalapeño Corn Biscuits**
1 teaspoon margarine
2 servings **Butternut Squash with Maple Glaze**
1 serving **Figs in a Chocolate Pool**
1 cup skim milk

2000 Calories — Day 8

Breakfast:

3 **Blintzes**
2 tablespoons non-fat yogurt
¾ cup blueberries

Snack:

1½ **Cinnamon Buns**
1 teaspoon margarine

Lunch:

¾ cup **Succotash Soup**
2 servings **Broccoli-Stuffed Potato**

Snack:

2½ cups watermelon cubes

Dinner:

1 serving **Pork Tenderloin with Chutney Glaze**
1½ cups baked acorn squash
1 teaspoon margarine
1 serving **Sautéed Radicchio and Watercress**
1 cup steamed cauliflower
1 **Butterscotch Square**
1 cup skim milk

2000 Calories — Day 9

Breakfast:

- ½ grapefruit
- 4 **Corn Pancakes**
- 1 teaspoon margarine
- 2 tablespoons low-calorie syrup

Snack:

- 2 small plums
- ¾ ounce unsalted pretzels

Lunch:

- ¾ cup **Creamy Orange Carrot Soup**
- 1 serving **White Bean Salad with Tomato Basil Vinaigrette**
- 1 whole wheat roll
- 1 teaspoon margarine
- 1 small apple

Snack:

- 1½ cups **Brandy Pumpkin Milk Shake**

Dinner:

- 4 ounces **Tandoori Chicken**
- 1 serving **Spinach Sag Paneer**
- 1 serving **Indian Curried Vegetables**
- 1 cup cooked brown rice
- 1 cup **Mocha Mousse**
- ¾ cup skim milk

2000 Calories — Day 10

Breakfast:

- 2 slices **Pumpkin Bread**
- 1 teaspoon margarine
- 2 teaspoons reduced-sugar jam
- ½ cup low-fat (1%) cottage cheese
- ½ cup **Apple Rhubarb Sauce**

Snack:

- ¾ cup cubed fresh pineapple
- ¾ cup non-fat yogurt

Lunch:

- 2 skewers **Beef Teriyaki**
- 1 cup cooked brown rice
- ¾ cup **Marinated Radishes**

Snack:

- 1½ cups **Minty Hot Chocolate**
- 4 **Poppy Seed Cookies with Raspberry Jam**

Dinner:

- 2 servings **Angel Hair with Scallops and Crabmeat**
- 1 serving **Broccoli with Anchovies**
- 2 tablespoons grated Parmesan cheese
- 1 whole wheat roll
- 1 teaspoon margarine
- 1 small salad
- 1 tablespoon **Honey Mustard Vinaigrette**
- ¾ cup **Raspberry Creme**

2000 Calories — Day 11

Breakfast:

1	cup cooked cereal
½	cup skim milk
1	small apple
1	slice pumpernickel toast
1	teaspoon margarine

Snack:

2	slices **Cranberry Nut Bread**
¾	cup skim milk

Lunch:

¾	cup **Sweet Potato Soup**
1½	servings **Fettuccine with Mushroom Stroganoff**
½	cup steamed broccoli
1	whole wheat roll
1	teaspoon margarine

Snack:

2	cups **Caramel Popcorn**
1	peach

Dinner:

1	serving **Chicken with Tarragon Sauce**
1	baked potato
1	teaspoon margarine
½	cup steamed green beans
1	small salad
1	tablespoon **Fresh Herb Vinaigrette**
1	serving **Peach Crisp**
1	cup skim milk

2000 Calories — Day 12

Breakfast:

1	serving **Poached Pears in Cranberry Glaze**
1	cup cooked oatmeal
1	cup skim milk
1	teaspoon margarine

Snack:

¾	cup **Mocha Shake**
1	**Applesauce Walnut Bran Muffin**

Lunch:

1½	cups **Six-Vegetable Chowder**
3	**Poppy Seed Biscuits**
1	teaspoon margarine
1	**Chili Rellenos**

Snack:

1	serving **Coffee-Flavored Root Beer Float**
2	ounces unsalted pretzels

Dinner:

4	ounces **Veal Loaf**
2	servings **Peppery Mushroom Sauce**
1	cup **Mashed Potatoes**
1	teaspoon margarine
1	serving **Zucchini Parmesan**
1	**Chocolate-Covered Banana**
½	cup skim milk

2000 Calories—Day 13

Breakfast:

- 4 **Blueberry Oatmeal Pancakes**
- 1 teaspoon margarine
- 3 tablespoons low-calorie syrup
- ⅓ cantaloupe

Snack:

- ¾ cup **Chocolate Mint Milk Shake**

Lunch:

- 1 cup **Vegetable Barley Soup**
- 1½ cups **Black Bean Confetti Salad**
- 1 baked potato
- 1 teaspoon margarine
- 1 **Rye Dinner Roll**

Snack:

- ⅔ cup **Fruity Couscous Pudding**
- ½ cup skim milk

Dinner:

- 1½ **Three-Herb Crab Cakes**
- 3 tablespoons **Tartar Sauce**
- 1 serving **Creamy Country Beets**
- ¾ cup steamed brussel sprouts
- 2 servings **Almost French-Fried Potatoes**
- 1 small salad
- 2 tablespoons **Sweet Orange Poppy Dressing**
- 1 serving **Pumpkin Pie**
- ¾ cup skim milk

2000 Calories—Day 14

Breakfast:

- 3-egg-white omelet
- ⅓ cup **Spicy Salsa**
- 1 **Homemade Flour Tortilla with Scallions**

Snack:

- 1 **Banana Walnut Muffin**
- 1 teaspoon margarine
- 1 cup skim milk

Lunch:

- 2 servings **Salmon-Stuffed Baked Potato**
- 1½ cups **Caesar Salad**
- ½ cup **Speckled Kasha**
- 1 whole wheat roll

- 1 teaspoon margarine
- 12 fresh cherries

Snack:

- 8 ounces **Piña Colada**

Dinner:

- ¾ cup **Cream of Broccoli Soup**
- 1 serving **Turkey-Stuffed Peppers**
- 2 5-inch ears of corn
- 1 serving **Caraway New Potatoes**
- 1 teaspoon margarine
- 1 small salad
- 1 tablespoon **Honey Mustard Vinaigrette**
- 1 slice **Strawberry Rhubarb Pie**

Solo Dining

(500-calorie dinners)

Meal 1:

1 serving **Broiled Grapefruit**
3 ounces **Broiled Ham with Orange Honey Glaze**
1 serving **Black Bean Confetti Salad**
1 serving **Tomato Okra Sauté**
1 small salad
1 tablespoon **Fresh Herb Vinaigrette**

Meal 2:

1 serving **Chili Rellenos**
1 whole **Mexican Pizza**
1 serving **Hot and Daring Zucchini Creole**
1 small corn on the cob
¾ cup **Mango Sorbet**

Meal 3:

2½ cups **Szechuan Stir-Fry**
1 cup cooked brown rice
1 orange, sliced

Meal 4:

3 ounces **Poached Salmon with Horseradish-Caper Sauce**
⅓ cup **Bulgur Pilaf with Basil and Pine Nuts**
1 serving **Double Mushroom Sauté with Tarragon**
1 whole wheat roll

Meal 5:

3 ounces **Pecan-Coated Chicken**
¾ cup **Turnip Greens with Smoked Clams**
1 serving **Baked Sweet Potatoes with Apples**
1 serving **Black-Eyed Peas with Tomatoes and Herbs**
1 **Orange Cream Pop**

Meal 6:

12 **Steamed Mussels in Herb Broth**
¾ cup **Lemon Couscous**
1 serving **Creamy Spinach**
Small salad
1 tablespoon **Honey Mustard Vinaigrette**

Meal 7:

½ **Artichoke with Tarragon Mustard Sauce**
1 serving **Pasta Tutti**
1 serving **Caesar Salad**
1 whole wheat roll
½ teaspoon margarine
½ cup steamed green beans

Lunches to Take to Work

(350-calorie lunches)

Lunch 1:

1 **Thai Salad with Spicy Dressing**
4 **Herbed Whole Wheat Bread Sticks**
1 orange

Lunch 2:

¾ cup **Salmon Salad** in pita bread
¾ cup strawberries

Lunch 3:

⅔ cup **Fruited Curried Chicken Salad**
2 slices whole wheat bread

Lunch 4:

1 **Chicken Tostada**
1 **Jalapeño Corn Biscuit**
½ teaspoon margarine
1 small green salad
1 tablespoon **Rosy Vinaigrette**

Lunch 5:

1 cup **Fish Chowder**
1 **Kasha Knish**
1 peach

Lunch 6:

8 ounces **Cold Creamy Cucumber Soup**
1 serving **Spicy Lemon Chicken Salad**
3 **Bagel Chips**
1 teaspoon margarine

Lunch 7:

¾ cup **Six-Vegetable Chowder**
1 serving **Ceviche with Chunky Vegetable Salsa**
1 **Homemade Flour Tortilla with Scallions**

Great Entertaining

The following menus give the amounts to cook for each party, as well as the amount to serve for weight control; "one serving" means that the cooked recipe divided among the number of guests yields the correct diet portion.

Winter Dinner for 8:

(500 calories per person)

	Prepare	Portion
French Onion Soup	1 recipe	¾ cup
Shrimp with Feta Cheese	double recipe	1 serving
Dilled Persian Rice	double recipe	⅓ cup
Savory Orange Carrots	double recipe	1 serving
Chocolate Meringue Cake	1 recipe	1 slice
Raspberry Sauce	1 recipe	¼ cup

Spring Dinner for 8:

(551 calories per person)

Artichokes with Mustard Tarragon Sauce	1 recipe	1 serving
Chicken Breasts Stuffed with Smoked Mozzarella and Basil	double recipe	1 serving
Broccoli with Anchovies	double recipe	1 serving
Fresh Berry Tart	1 recipe	1 piece

Summer Dinner for 8:

(587 calories per person)

Cream of Broccoli Soup	1 recipe	¾ cup
Poached Chicken Salad with Raspberry Vinaigrette	double recipe	1 serving
Poppy Seed Biscuits	1½ recipes	2 biscuits
Margarine		1 teaspoon
Strawberry Rhubarb Pie	1 recipe	1 slice

Fall Dinner for 4:

(593 calories per person)

Salmon Wrapped in Phyllo	1 recipe	1 serving
Wild and Brown Rice	1 recipe	⅓ cup
Boston Bibb Salad with Roquefort and Apples	1 recipe	1 serving
Rye Dinner Rolls	1 recipe	1 roll
Poached Pears in Cranberry Glaze	1 recipe	1 serving

Brunch for 8:

(467 calories per person)

Crustless Spinach Mushroom Quiche	1 recipe	2 slices
Spinach Salad with Smoked Oysters and Orange Vinaigrette Dressing	double recipe	1 serving
Bulgur Pilaf with Basil and Pine Nuts	1 recipe	⅓ cup
Cranberry Nut Bread	1 recipe	1 slice
Exotic Fresh Fruits with Mango Cream	1 recipe	1 serving

Open House Hors d'Oeuvres for 20:

(312 calories per person)

Spicy Tomato Juice		1 drink
Beef Teriyaki	1 recipe	1 skewer
Vegetable Terrine	1 recipe	1 slice
Bagel Chips	double recipe	1 chip
California Nori Rolls	1 recipe	1 piece
Futomaki	1 recipe	1 piece
White Pizza with Broccoli and Anchovies	1 recipe	1 piece
Spicy Cocktail Balls with	1 recipe	1 ball
Sweet and Sour Tomato Sauce	1 recipe	

Barbecue for 4:

(482 calories per person)

Barbecued Chicken Legs	1 recipe	3 legs
Creamy Cole Slaw	½ recipe	½ cup
Pear and Potato Salad	½ recipe	½ cup
Sweet Potato Biscuits	1 recipe	1 biscuit
Watermelon		1 slice

Picnic for 8:

(481 calories per person)

Poached Salmon with Horseradish-Caper Sauce	double recipe	3 ounces
Penne with Basil and Sweet Peppers	double recipe	¾ cup
Creamy Cucumbers and Onions	1 recipe	¾ cup
Poppy Seed Biscuits	1 recipe	1 biscuit
Chocolate Brownies	1 recipe	1 piece

Picnic for 8:

(491 calories per person)

Vegetarian Spring Rolls with Hot and Spicy Dipping Sauce	1 recipe	2 pieces
Orzo Salad	1 recipe	½ cup
Indonesian Chicken Satay	double recipe	4 ounces
Poppy Seed Cookies with Raspberry Jam	1½ recipe	2 cookies
Cubed fresh pineapple		¾ cup

Index